Anesthetic considerations for elderly Eisenmenger syndrome

Authors: Hala M Goma ,MD ,P rofessor Of Anesthesia,cairo University.

Email:

ahmeda1995@yahoo.com

Table of contents

Abstract

Only 15–25% of congenital heart disease patients survive into adulthood. Approximately 90% of these children survive to adulthood due to Advances in prenatal diagnosis, interventional cardiology; pediatric cardiac surgery, anesthesia, and critical care have resulted in survival of **Eisenmenger syndrome.** **Eisenmenger syndrome** is defined as the process in which a left to right shunt caused by a congenital heart defect in the fetal heart causes increased flow through the pulmonary vasculature, causing pulmonary hypertension, which in turn causes increased pressures in the right side of the heart, and reversal of the shunt into a right. Eisenmenger syndrome is a cyanotic heart defect characterized by a long-standing intracardiac shunt (caused by ventricular septal defect, atrial septal defect, or less commonly, patent ductus arteriosus. The long term survival of patients of **Eisenmenger** syndrome will make challenge for anesthetist; the risk during anesthesia of **Eisenmenger** syndrome may be increased. Combination of anesthetic considerations of Eisenmenger syndrome and anesthetic management of elderly patients must be considered. In Eisenmenger syndrome there is pulmonary hypertension lung congestion and increase risk of pneumonia. In elderly non cardiac patients there is increased risk of COPD, pneumonia; sleep apnea conduction abnormalities, bradyarrythmias and hypertension are very common among the elderly, Decreased renal blood flow and kidney mass decrease with age with increased risk of renal impairment due to long standing Eisenmenger syndrome. This book contains the practical anesthetic considerations for anesthesia elderly Eisenmenger syndrome.

Introduction

Only 15–25% of congenital heart disease patients survive into adulthood. Approximately 90% of these children survive to adulthood due to Advances in prenatal diagnosis, interventional cardiology; pediatric cardiac surgery, anesthesia, and critical care have resulted in survival of.

Eisenmenger syndrome (or **ES**, **Eisenmenger reaction** or **tardive cyanosis**) is defined as the process in which a left to right shunt caused by a congenital heart defect in the fetal heart causes increased flow through the pulmonary vasculature, causing pulmonary hypertension, which in turn causes increased pressures in the right side of the heart and reversal of the shunt into a right. Eisenmenger syndrome is a cyanotic heart defect characterized by a long-standing intracardiac shunt (caused by ventricular septal defect, atrial septal defect, or less commonly, patent ductus arteriosus.

Sign and symptoms of Eisenmenger syndrome

1. Cyanosis
2. High red blood cell count
3. Swollen or clubbed finger tips (clubbing)
4. Fainting (also known as syncope).
5. Heart failure.
6. Abnormal heart rhythms.
7. Bleeding disorders.
8. Coughing up blood.
9. Iron deficiency.
10. Infections (endocarditis and pneumonia).
11. Kidney problems.
12. Stroke.
13. Gout due to increased uric acid resorption and production with impaired excretion.
14. Gallstones.

Complications of Eisenmenger syndrome are

- fainting spell,
- thromboembolism,
- Hypovolemia.

The long term survival of patients of **Eisenmenger** syndrome will make challenge for anesthetics; the risk during anesthesia of **Eisenmenger** syndrome may be increased. Combination of anesthetic considerations of Eisenmenger syndrome and anesthetic management of elderly patients must be considered.

Long term cardiac complications of congenital heart disease:

Pulmonary hypertension may be caused by pulmonary venous hypertension secondary to elevated ventricular end diastolic pressure, elevated pulmonary venous atrial pressure, or pulmonary vein stenosis.

Ventricular dysfunction:

Common causes of heart failure in Eisenmenger syndrome are coronary artery disease including a previous myocardial infarction (heart attack), high blood pressure, atrial fibrillation, valvular heart disease, excess alcohol use, infection, and cardiomyopathy of an unknown cause.

Dysrhythmias

- Atrial tachyarrhythmias are often resistant to pharmacological treatment and can result in rapid hemodynamic deterioration.
- Ventricular dysrhythmias are most frequently encountered in patients who have significantly decreased right or left ventricular function.
- Other risk factors include previous ventriculotomy, earlier surgical era, or older age at initial surgery.

Geriatric cardiovascular pathophysiological changes:

- Decreased beta-adrenergic responsiveness and they have an increased incidence of conduction abnormalities, bradyarrythmias and hypertension.
- Fibrotic infiltration of cardiac conduction pathways make the elderly patient vulnerable to conduction delay and to atrial and ventricular ectopy
- Elderly patients also have an increased reliance on Frank-Starling mechanism for cardiac output. It is therefore important to consider fluid administration carefully.
- In the non compliant older heart, small changes in venous return will produce large changes in ventricular preload and cardiac output. Due to diastolic dysfunction and decreased vascular compliance, the elderly patient compensates poorly for hypovolemia. Similarly, exaggerated transfusion is also poorly tolerated.

Pulmonary anesthetic considerations of elderly Eisenmenger syndrome

- In Eisenmenger syndrome there is pulmonary hypertension lung congestion and increase risk of pneumonia
- In elderly non cardiac patients there are increased risk of COPD, pneumonia, sleep apnea are very common among the elderly.
- Closing volume increases with age, and FEV1 declines 8-10% per decade due to reduced pulmonary compliance. PaO2 decreases progressively with age because of V/Q mismatch and anatomical shunt .All these pathophysiological changes may increase respiratory complications of Eisenmenger syndrome.
- The chest X-Ray shows the heart position (Dextrocardia) and size, atelectasis, acute respiratory infection, vascular markings and elevated hemidiaphragm. Patients with diminished pulmonary blood flow show reduced pulmonary markings.

Noncardiac complications of long standing Eisenmenger syndrome:

1. Secondary erythrocytosis.
2. Gall bladder stones.
3. Renal impairment.

4. Developmental abnormalities.
5. Central nervous abnormalities, such as seizure disorders from previous thromboembolic events or cerebrovascular accidents, hearing or visual loss.
6. Restrictive and obstructive lung disease.
7. Uncontrolled bleeding due to damaged capillaries and high pressure.
8. Clots due to hyper viscosity and stasis of blood .coagulation defects which may interfere with regional anesthesia.
9. Coughing hemoptysis, bleeding may lead to iron deficiency anemia

Pathophysiology of the renal function due to aging:

- Decreased renal blood flow and kidney mass decrease with age.

- Serum creatinine level remains stable due to a reduction in muscle tissue.

- Impairment of sodium handling, concentrating ability and diluting capacity predisposes elderly patients to dehydration and fluid overload.

- Reduced renal blood flow and decreased nephrons mass increase the risk of acute renal failure in the postoperative period.

  Eisenmenger syndrome has renal problems:

  - Increase risk of renal impairment when accompanied especially with the pathophysiological changes in elderly patients.

  There are major risk factors in surgery for an elderly Eisenmenger syndrome patient

  1. Renal hypoperfusion as a consequence of systemic hypotension,

  2. Hypovolemia,

  3. Cardiac dysfunction.

Preoperative Management

Aim of Preoperative Evaluation:

1. **Determination of the risk factors.**
2. **Determination of the cediac condition is stable so no further cardiac testing is needed.**
3. Specialized cardiac testing, echocardiography or cardiac catheterization is needed.
4. Decompensated heart failure, cardio logical consultation reference is required for proper control.
5. The need for anticoagulant.
6. Control of diabetes, hypertension.
7. Old age may be assessed for carotid end areterectomy, especially before major operations.
8. Evaluation of the nutritional status, correction of anemia, and hypo albuminia.
9. Preoperative renal assessment and base line parameters are estimated for post operative comparison

Preoperative risk
- Poor functional class.
- Pulmonary hypertension.
- Congestive heart failure.
- Cyanosis.
- Major surgery and procedures that involve one lung ventilation
- Changes in position (*e.g.* , prone, Trendelenburg) could produce important hemodynamic effects.

Preoperative evaluation of cardiac function

Cardiac function   assessment:

- Evaluation and Care for Noncardiac Surgery have been published by the American Heart Association and American College of Cardiology (2007)
- . Individual cardiac evaluation must take into account active cardiac conditions, functional capacity, additional clinical risk factors and surgical risk.
- Stable, asymptomatic patients with normal functional capacity can proceed to elective anesthesia and surgery without further cardiac evaluation.
- Active cardiac conditions require evaluation and treatment by a cardiology service prior to elective surgery.

- Established indicated beta blocker and statin medication is to be continued; timely institution of beta blocker medication (target heart rate, < 65 bpm) may be required depending on the risk of surgery,

- There is inadequate evidence at present to define the optimal time course for acute beta-blockade, or the groups of patients in whom preoperative beta-blockade should be initiated in the absence of contraindications. Nevertheless, addition of beta-blockers to the preoperative regimen should be considered in patients with evidence of or at risk for coronary disease undergoing major surgery. There is also evidence that long-term beta-adrenoceptor or calcium channel blockade or nitrate therapy for the high-risk cardiac patient offers little protection against silent myocardial ischemia, nonfatal infarction, cardiac failure and cardiac death.
- Elective surgery should be postponed in patients with signs and symptoms of cardiac failure for optimization. Patient may require digoxin, diuretics and inotropes. Mechanical ventilation may be necessary for pulmonary edema.

History and physical examination :

- Exercise tolerance.
- Angina pectoris.
- Myocardial infarction

- Coexisting disease, as diabetes mellitus, hypertension. Chronic obstructive pulmonary disease in patients with history of cigarette smoking.
- Current medications- like beta blockers.
- Calcium channel blockers, nitrates should be continued until the morning of surgery. Patient may be on oral anticoagulants or aspirin which should be stopped 5-7 days prior to surgery.

Cerbro vascular accident history due to:

1. **Increased risk of thromboembolism in Eisenmenger syndrome.**
2. **Elderly may have prolonged hypertension disease, atherosclerosis, thrombo embolic stroke and the need for coagulation.**

Preoperative testing:
- **Complete blood picture for if there is polycythemia with Eisenmenger syndrome, platelets count, .thrombo cytosis**
- **Coagulation profile, prothrombin concentration, INR level.**
- **Renal function, creatinine, electrolyte levels.**
- **Liver functions, albumin, bilirubin level, ALT, AST levels.**

Specialized cardiac testing:

- **ECG, echocardiography ejection fraction, any valvular lesion , wall mo-tion abnormalities, LV function and pressure gradients,**
- **Holter monitoring, Treadmill test, thallium scintig-raphy to detect myocardium at risk, radionuclide ven-triculography,**
- **dobutamine stress test(DST) for evaluating inducible ischemia in patients who have poor functional capacity**
- **Coronary angiography.**
- **Decompensated heart failure:**

Heart failure (HF) is a risk factor for cardiac complications after noncardiac surgery:

After major surgery, chronic stable HF is associated with two- to threefold higher 30-day mortality and hospital readmission compared with coronary artery disease.

Risk factors lead to acute heart failure should be avoided during anesthesia:

- Myocardial ischemia or infarction.
- Worsening of cardiac valve dysfunction.
- Atrial fibrillation and other arrhythmias.
- Cardio toxic agents.
- Stress-induced (Takotsubo) cardiomyopathy.
- Rapid progression of underlying chronic HF.
- Severe hypertension.
- Renal failure.
- Pulmonary emboli.

Implantable cardioverter defibrillators and pacemakers:
Cardiac pacemakers are effective treatments for of bradyarrhythmias. it provides an appropriate heart rate and heart rate response, cardiac pacing can reestablish effective circulation and more normal hemodynamics that are compromised by a slow heart rate

Management decisions for permanent pacemaker implantation are the following clinical factors:
- ●The association of symptoms with a bradyarrhythmia
- ●The location of the conduction abnormality
  Risk factors for hospitalization of paced patients

- The anesthetist should understand both the normal patterns of pacemaker and implantable cardioverter defibrillator usage.
- Electromagnetic interference, Surgical cautery in hospital.
- The clinician must be prepared to intervene in an appropriate manner to prevent patient injury.

Factors affecting the perioperative management:

1. Individualized to the patient.
2. The type of CIED.
3. The procedure being performed.

A CIED team:

The physicians and physician are the extenders who monitor the CIED function of the patient.

Role of CIED team:

- Communication with the surgical or procedural team to identify the type of procedure and the risk.
- Prescription for the perioperative management of patients with CIEDs.
- review of the records of the CIED clinic.
- consultation from CIED specialists if the information is not available.

According to (The Heart Rhythm Society (HRS)/American Society of Anesthesiologists (ASA) Expert Consensus Statement on the Perioperative Management of Patients with Implantable Defibrillators, Pacemakers and Arrhythmia Monitors: Facilities and Patient Management: Executive Summary Heart Rhythm, Vol 8, No 7, July 2011)

Essential elements of the information given to the CIED physician

- Type of procedure.
- Anatomic location of surgical procedure
- Patient position during the procedure.
- Will monopolar electrosurgery be used.
- Will cardioversion or defibrillation be used
- Surgical venue (operating room, procedure suite, etc.)
- Anticipated postprocedural arrangements (anticipated discharge to home "23 hours, inpatient admission to critical care bed, telemetry bed).
- Cardiothoracic or chest wall surgical procedure that could impair/damage or encroach upon the CIED leads.
- Anticipated large blood loss.
- Operation in close proximity to CIED.

Essential elements of the pre-operative CIED evaluation

- Date of last device interrogation.
- Type of device—Pacemaker, ICD, CRT-D, CRT-P, ILR,
- Implantable hemodynamic monitor
- Manufacturer and model
- Indication for device: - Pacemaker: e.g., sick sinus syndrome, AV block, syncope - ICD: primary or secondary prevention - Cardiac resynchronization therapy •
- Battery longevity documented as #3 months.
- the leads less than 3 months old
- Programming - Pacing mode and programmed lower rate.
- Lowest heart rate for shock delivery.
- Lowest heart rate for ATP delivery.
- Rate responsive sensor type.
- Is the patient pacemaker dependent and what is the underlying rhythm and heart rate if can be determined.
- the response of this device to magnet placement.
- Magnet pacing rate for a PM.
- Pacing amplitude response to magnet function.
- Will ICD detections resume automatically with removal of the magnet? Does this device allow for magnet application function to be disabled? If so, document programming of patient's device for this feature. •
- Any alert status on CIED generator or lead.
- Last pacing threshold— document adequate safety margin with the date of that threshold

Cardiac monitoring interactions with CIEDs

- Over counting the heart rate due to counting pacemaker spikes and QRS complexes individually.

- Inability to identify pacemaker spikes with monitors employing high frequency filters falsely "marking" artifact as a pacemaker spike.
- Pacemaker initiated heart rate increase due to rate responsive pacemaker algorithms with inappropriate response by surgical team –
- Most rate sensors employ an accelerometer such that patient movement could increase the patient's paced rate if the sensor is not inactivated.
- Minute ventilation creates a unique situation where current emitted by the CIED to measure changes in thoracic impedance can be detected by monitoring equipment and appears to be rapid pacing without capture.

Perioperative Management of Patients With Devices:
- Defibrillation patches should be placed if the patient is at high risk for ventricular arrhythmias or with extensive surgical procedures.
- Emergency equipment should be easily accessible to the procedure area.
- The electrosurgical units must be properly grounded.
- Although adverse interactions with contemporary earth-grounded electrosurgical systems are uncommon.
- Problems can occur if not grounded properly. Optimal "grounding" involves the use of a split foil return electrode, which allows for detection of proper application to the patient..
- The return electrode should be placed such that the current is directed away from the CIED.

Recommendations for the intraoperative monitoring of patients with CIEDs

- External defibrillation equipment is required in the OR and immediately available for all patients with pacemakers or ICDs having surgical and sedation procedures or procedures where EMI may occur.
- All patients with ICDs deactivated should be on a cardiac monitor and during surgery should have immediate availability of defibrillation.
- Some patients may need to have pads placed prophylactically during surgery (e.g., high risk patients and patients in whom pad placement will be difficult due to surgical site.
- All patients with pacemakers or ICDs require plethysmographic or arterial pressure monitoring for all surgical and sedation procedures.
- Use an ECG monitor with a pacing mode set to recognize pacing stimuli.
- PMs may be made asynchronous as needed with either a magnet application or reprogramming provided that the pulse generator is accessible.
- ICD detection may be suspended by either magnet application as needed or reprogramming, provided that the pulse generator is accessible.
- During the placement of central lines using the Seldinger technique from the upper body, caution should be exercicised to avoid causing false detections and/or shorting the RV coil to the SVC coil.
- Increased risk of thromboembolism inpatient of Eisenmenger syndrome.
- Because of interactions with monitoring, ventilation, and other impedance monitoring operative devices, inactivating minute ventilation sensors can be considered.
- Keep a magnet immediately available for all patients with a CIED who are undergoing a procedure that may involve EMI.

Anesthetic considerations of thromboembolism

- Venous thromboembolism due to Deep venous thrombosis and then pulmonary embolism. Heparin and low-molecular-weight heparin followed by oral anticoagulation with vitamin K agonists is the first line and current accepted standard therapy with good efficacy. However, there is significant risk of bleeding and drug, food and disease interactions that require frequent monitoring.
- New oral coagulants used:
  Dabigatran, rivaroxaban, apixaban, and edoxaban are the novel oral anticoagulants that are available for use in stroke prevention in atrial fibrillation and for the treatment and prevention of venous thromboembolism. They are Xa inhibitors
- The Xa inhibitors have interactions with medications that affect the CYP3A4 and beta glycoprotein

Drugs should be avoided with these drugs are

1. Drugs increase risk of bleeding heparin and warfarin
2. Drugs decrease effects Phenobarbital and dexamethasone
3. Dose reduction with Drugs increase coagulation as Amiodaron, propanolo,verapamil,nicardipin,erythromycin
4. Used cautiously with Antiplatltes, nonsteroidal anti-inflammatory which increase anticoagulant effect.
5. Drugs Decrease anti coagulant effect as Antiacid, H2 blocker and proton pump inhibitors.

- The American Academy of Orthopaedic Surgeons (AAOS) published guidelines in 2007 for the prevention of symptomatic PE in patients undergoing total joint replacement (www.aaos.org/guidelines.pdf).
- These evidence-based guidelines allowed assignment of the patient to 1 of 4 categories (based on risk of PE and bleeding) and differed from those of the ACCP. The major deviations from ACCP guidelines are as follows:
  (1) Mechanical prophylaxis should be used in all patients,
  (2) Warfarin is a suitable alternative in all categories.

(3) In patients in whom there is an increased risk for bleeding, regardless of the risk of PE, prophylactic options include warfarin, aspirin, or mechanical prophylaxis only.

- Antithrombotic therapy may be safely interrupted until adequate surgical hemostasis is achieved.
- Bridging anticoagulation with unfractionated or LMWH is required until the time of surgery (and reinitiated in the immediate postoperative period). It may also be necessary to postpone elective surgeries in patients where a suitable "bridge" has not been identified and antithrombotic therapy is critical; premature discontinuation of dual antiplatelet therapy in patients with coronary stents has been associated with stent thrombosis, myocardial infarction and death.
- The initial recommendations in 1986 by the American College of Chest Physicians (ACCP) stated that patients undergoing hip arthroplasty receive dextran, adjusted-dose standard heparin (approximately 3500 U every 8 hrs), warfarin (started 48 hrs postoperatively to achieve a prothrombin time [PT] 1.25–1.5 times baseline), or dextran plus intermittent pneumatic compression (IPC).
- The highest risk for thromboembolism and receive prophylaxis with low-molecular weight heparin (LMWH), fondaparinux (2.5 mg started 6-24 hrs postoperatively) or warfarin (started before or after operation with a mean target international normalized ratio [INR] of 2.5).
- However, adjusted-dose heparin, dextran, and venous foot pumps are no longer recommended as sole methods of thromboprophylaxis, although IPC is considered appropriate for patients at a high risk for bleeding. Importantly, the duration of thromboprophylaxis is continued after hospital discharge for a total of 10 to 35 days.
- In general, LMWH thromboprophylaxis is still not considered a contraindication to epidural anesthesia/analgesia in Europe.

Complications during usage of anticoagulants

- Spinal hematoma, defined as symptomatic bleeding within the spinal neuraxis, is a rare and potentially catastrophic complication of spinal or epidural anesthesia

- Hemorrhage into the spinal canal most commonly occurs in the epidural space, most likely because of the prominent epidural venous plexus, although anesthetic variables, such as needle size and catheter placement, may also affect the site of clinically significant bleeding

Risk factors for spinal hematoma

1. Old Age

2. Female Sex

3. Ankolsing spondylitis or spinal stenosis

4. Traumatic needle,

5. Catheter placement

6. Epidural more than spinal

7. Placement of epidural catheter during LMWH administration

8. Immediate preoperative or intraoperative LMWH

9. Early postoperatively LMWH

10. Repeated doses of heparin

11. Antiplatelts or non steroidal drugs

Preoperative medications for noncardiac surgery of Eisenmenger syndrome

Anxiolytics and hypnotics must be undertaken very cautiously because hypoventilation and hypercapnia may produce deleterious increases in pulmonary vascular resistance.

Endocarditis Prophylaxis

The American Heart Association has recently published updated guidelines for the prevention of infective endocarditis, they stated that only patients with cardiac conditions

- patients with previous endocarditis,
- unrepaired cyanotic CHD,
- palliative shunts and conduits;
- completely repaired congenital heart defects with prosthetic material or device, whether placed by surgery or by catheter intervention, during the first 6 months after the procedure;
- Repaired CHD with residual defects at the site or adjacent to the site of a prosthetic patch or prosthetic device (which inhibit endothelialization).

All cardiac medications should be continued up to and including the morning of surgery with the exception of anticoagulation involving warfarin, and perhaps large doses of angiotensin converting enzyme inhibitors and angiotensin II receptor antagonists in patients with hypertension or heart failure.

Intraoperative management:

Intraoperative risk during anesthesia of Eisenmenger syndrome

Eisenmenger syndrome is one of the leading causes of perioperative death (up to 19%) in patients undergoing non cardiac surgery (NCS). Cardiac arrest and pulmonary hypertensive crisis

- urgency,
- duration of surgery,
- Anesthesia used and underlying pathology.
- Profound hemodynamic variability such as heart rate, blood pressure, volume status, oxygenation, and neurohormonal activation adds an extra stress on an already abnormal cardiopulmonary system.
- Hematocrit >60%, arterial oxygen saturation <80%, right ventricular hypertension, syncopal attack and a fixed pulmonary hypertension not responsive to oxygen carries poor prognosis.
- bleeding due to platelet dysfunction, thrombosis due to Polcythemia,
- paradoxical embolism and arrhythmia

Hemodynamic monitoring

The goal is to detect sudden changes in hemodynamics very early so as to initiate appropriate treatment and prevent further complications

- All IV lines are a potential source of systemic embolization and should have filters placed along them. Furthermore,
- Pulse oximeter can provide continuous monitoring of the degree of ven-arterial mixing.
- Periodic arterial blood gas for assessment of acidosis, hypercarbia and hypoxia, which can increase the pulmonary vascular resistance and increase right to left shunting.
- Arterial line Continuous intra-arterial monitoring of the blood pressure is a safe and reliable means of early recognition of sudden alterations in intravascular volume and haemodynamics.
- Central venous line or pulmonary artery pressure recording.

- Periodic arterial blood gas determination if desired.
- The pulmonary artery catheter can also provide critical information, but the benefit should be balanced against the risk of complications from insertion and as pulmonary artery rupture.
- ventricular arrhythmias, pulmonary embolization, plus the additional risk of infection and paradoxical embolism
- In addition cardiac output measurement by thermo dilution technique can be spurious .
- Patients undergoing intermediate to high-risk procedures might warrant placement of a pulmonary artery catheter (with or without oximetry)
- They are polycythaemic, intra-arterial catheterization may be associated with a higher incidence of post-cannulation thrombus formation.
- Insertion of central venous catheters has the potential risks of infection and paradoxical air embolus.
- The use of intra-arterial monitoring in all patients with the Eisenmenger syndrome as hypotension, unless immediately corrected, will allow the intracardiac shunt to become wholly from right to left, with disastrous consequences.
- A cent`ral venous catheter, although not mandatory, should be considered.

Intraoperative Anesthetic management:

Anesthetic management of an elderly **Eisenmenger** syndrome should include participation of anesthesiologists, cardiologists, intensivists, and surgeons.

Golden role during anesthesia of Eisenmenger syndrome
- An increase in central venous return, in the presence of a high, fixed pulmonary vascular resistance, would increase the right-to-left shunt, whilst a decrease in venous return would decrease pulmonary and systemic blood flow, both conditions resulting in hypoxemia.

Choice of anesthetic technique

Goals of suitable anesthetic technique

A. **Anesthetic management for cardiac problem:**

21

1. Avoid increase pulmonary pressure.

2. Avoid volume over load.

3. Light anesthesia and patchy regional anesthesia, can lead to increase the systemic vascular resistance, increased after load leads to ventricular failure.

4. Maintenance of adequate filling pressure.

5. Optimal analgesia.

6. Management of clinical deterioration.

B. Renal protection for Eisenmenger syndrome undergo non cardiac operation

- Euvolemia by perioperative monitoring.

- Manipulation of oxygen delivery by volume expansion.

- Inotropic drugs may decrease mortality in surgical patients from postoperative renal dysfunction.

- Correction of intraoperative anemia secondary to intraoperative bleeding

- Careful monitoring of urine output CVP (central venous pressure to adjust proper hydration, and avoidance of fluid over load.

- Higher molecular weight hydroxyethylene starch (hetastarch and pentastarch MW ≥ 200 kDa) should be avoided in patients with severe sepsis due to an increased risk of AKI.

Definition of post operative renal dysfunction:

RIFLE classification (increase in SCr at least 50% from preoperative value and/or a reduction in urine output 0.5mLkg1 hr 1 for 6 hours)

Contributing factors for General versus regional anesthesia:

I. **Anesthesia and elderly patients:**

1. Dosage requirements for local and general anesthetics are reduced.

2. Administration of a given volume of epidural anesthetic results in a more cephalic spread, having though a shorter duration of sensory and motor block.

3. Elderly patients take more time to recover from general anesthesia especially if they were disoriented perioperatively, however there is a risk of thromboembolism and stroke in Eisenmenger syndrome Geriatric patients experience varying degrees of delirium. They are sensitive to centrally acting anticholinergic agents.

4. The incidence of delirium is less with regional anesthesia, provided that there is no additional sedation.

5. The circulating level of albumin which is the main plasma binding protein for acidic drugs decreases with age.

6. On the other hand, the level of α-1 acid glycoprotein the binding protein for basic drugs increases. The effect of aging on pharmacokinetic depends upon the drug is used.

7. The decrease in total body water leads to a reduction in the central compartment and increased serum concentrations after a bolus administration of a drug. On the other hand, the increase in body fat results in a greater volume of distribution, thus prolonging drug action.

8. Drug metabolism could probably be altered by the aging effect on hepatic or renal function.

9. The elderly are more sensitive to anesthetic agents and generally require smaller doses for the same clinical effect, and drug action is usually prolonged.

General versus regional anesthesia for Eisenmenger syndrome

- Whether general or regional anesthesia the aim is the Balance between SVR and PVR is essential in the anaesthetic management of patient with shunts. Blood flow through shunt depends upon diameter of defect and balance between systemic and vascular resistance

- General anesthesia is preferred by most anaesthetists due to fear of reduced SVR by regional anesthesia.
- Regional anesthesia can be used but SVR should be maintained at all cost. Monitoring of ventricular and supraventricular tachycardia in the postoperative phase and keep them in ICU.

Technique for neuraxial anesthesia

- Epidural anesthesia has been successfully employed for minor surgeries such as tubal ligation and cesarean section.
- The resulting sympathetic blockade and decrease in both preload and afterload may be very hazardous, general anesthesia is preferable for these patients.

Technique for general anesthesia:

Induction

Hypotension is more common in patients with Eisenmenger syndrome when a vasopressor is not used during the peri-induction period, regardless of induction agent. The use of a vasopressor is recommended. Intra cardiac shunts prolong inhalation induction while IV induction is faster. R-L shunt reversal occur when SVR drops or PVR increases.

- Opioid as short-acting, intravenous (IV as fentanyl, which is usually well tolerated.
- Low-dose induction agent such as sodium thiopental or Ketamine.
- Etomidate tended to have better hemodynamic stability than other induction agents.
- Recommendations for anesthesiologists to use of a vasopressor before or during induction to reduce hypotension.
- complete avoidance of inhalational induction
- Intra cardiac shunts prolong inhalation induction while IV induction is faster. R-L shunt (e.g. TOF) or shunt reversal occur when SVR drops or PVR increases.

Maintenance

- inhalational agent, for example, isoflurane

- Atracurium and vecuronium can be used as muscle relaxants because of their minimal effects on the cardiovascular system.
- Limit the use of inhalation anesthetics due to associated myocardial depression. Maintain normal sinus rhythm and preload during anesthesia.
- After load reduction by vasodilators may be required in many situations to reduce cardiac workload and improve cardiac output.

  Factors increase decrease pulmonary blood flow:

  - Systemic vascular resistance,
  - Intermittent positive pressure ventilation can decrease pulmonary blood flow and hence increase the right-to-left shunt
  - normal tidal volumes are used with minimal inflation pressures,
  - High intrathoracic pressures must be avoided.
  - Lumley, Morgan and Sykes commended minute volumes of 5-8 liters per minute with tidal volumes of 5.5-6 ml/kg body weight to maintain $PaCO_2$ within normal limits in adults. The most suitable muscle relaxants are those with minimal effects on the cardiovascular system.

  Avoidance of Hypoxemia:
  - Inadequate pulmonary blood flow and/or admixture of deoxygenated with oxygenated blood in systemic circulation. These patients are polycythaemic, . Dehydration should be avoided, maintenance of systemic blood pressure, minimizing additional resistance to pulmonary blood flow and avoid sudden increase in oxygen demand (crying, struggling, and inadequate level of anaesthesia).
  - Hypercyanotic spell under anaesthesia responds to volume, Increase SVR with alpha agonists such as Phenylephrine and decreasing right ventricular outflow track obstruction with beta blockade.

Management of polycythemia

Hyper viscosity will disappear after adequate phlebotomy within 24 hours resulting in increased cardiac output and systemic blood flow due to decreased whole blood viscosity and decreased systemic vascular resistance

There are two indications for phlebotomies:

1. moderate to severe hyper viscosity symptoms due to secondary erythrocytosis;
2. Preoperative phlebotomy for autologous blood donation if the hematocrit level is above 65%.

- Intravenous fluid should be administered in preoperative fasting phase to avoid hypotension episodes.
- Avoidance of increased Rt to Lt shunts

Factors increased pulmonary pressure:

Hypothermia

Stress

Pain

Acidosis

Hypercarbia

Hypoxia

Elevated intrathoracic pressure

The Pathophysiology of pulmonary hypertension in patients with Eisenmenger syndrome

It is associated with a neurohormonal imbalance of endogenous pulmonary vasodilators and vasoconstrictors. This imbalance leads to vascular remodeling, intimal fibrosis, and increased pulmonary vascular resistance (PVR). Therefore, in the management of patients with Eisenmenger syndrome, the use of pulmonary vasodilating agents that have been shown to be useful in the management of patients with IPAH is conceptually appealing; data support this use.

Prostacyclin

Long-term prostacyclin therapy was shown to improve hemodynamics (decrease in mean pulmonary artery pressure, improvement in cardiac index, and decrease in PVR) and the quality of life in patients with congenital heart disease and pulmonary arterial hypertension (PAH).

Epoprostenol

a continuous intravenous infusion via a central catheter because of its short half-life (5 min). Patients must carry a portable pump in a waist pack and must maintain the drug at a cool temperature during the infusion. This therapy is extremely expensive It has been shown to improve pulmonary pressure, 6MWT distance, oxygenation, and quality of life in patients.

Treprostinil

It is a prostacyclin analogue that is administered by continuous subcutaneous infusion. its use in children with pulmonary hypertension .

Iloprost is an inhaled prostacyclin administered intermittently 6-9 times daily via nebulizer and is approved for adults with IPAH.

Endothelin receptor antagonists

Bosentan, an endothelin receptor antagonist that has been approved for patients with IPAH, was the second vasodilator to be evaluated in patients with Eisenmenger syndrome.

Ambrisentan, which has been approved for IPAH, is a specific endothelium receptor-1 type A antagonist. Data on its use in Eisenmenger syndrome are limited.

Phosphodiesterase inhibitors

Sildanfil, another vasodilatory agent, was originally used for erectile dysfunction but has since been approved by the US Food and Drug Administration (FDA) for IPAH. It acts as an inhibitor of phosphodiesterase 5, resulting in an increase in cyclic guanosine monophosphate (cGMP) and vascular relaxation. It works synergistically with inhaled nitric oxide.

Nitric oxide replacement

Innovative home nitric oxide delivery devices have been described and have been used on a compassionate basis in patients with severe pulmonary hypertension.

management for arrhythmia

mechanism of action of anti arrythemic drugs

Receptor Class2 Drugs Na+ , K+ channels IA

Procainamide, quinidine, amiodarone

Na+ channels IB

Lidocaine, phenytoin, *mexiletine, *tocainide

Beta adrenoceptors II

Esmolol, amiodarone, propranolol, atenolol, *sotalol

K+ channels III

Bretylium, ibutilide, *sotalol, *dofetilide

Ca2+ channels IV

Verapamil, diltiazem, amiodarone

Management of perioperative arrhythmia

a) **Reversible causes of supraventricular tachycardia and nonsustained ventricular tachycardia.**

These conditions are usually reversible.

1. Hypoxaemia
2. Hypercarbia
3. Acidosis

4. Hypotension
5. Electrolyte imbalances
6. Mechanical irritation
7. Pulmonary artery catheter
8. Chest tube
9. Hypothermia
10. Adrenergic stimulation (light anaesthesia)
11. Proarrhythmic drugs Micro/macro shock
12. Cardiac ischemia
13. Management of supra ventricular tachycardia

b) Indications of DC cardioversion

The aim is to prevent the life-threatening complications of hypoperfusion, such as central nervous system or cardiac ischemia.

   i.   Patients with narrow complex tachycardia who are dangerously Hypotensive

  ii.   cardiac ischemia

          c) A systolic pressure below 80 mm Hg requires immediate synchronous cardioversion.

.Pharmacological management

Adenosine may be administered as a 6 mg i.v. bolus (repeated with 12 mg if no response).

Esmolol

It is largely b1-receptor selective and is generally well tolerated by patients with chronic obstructive lung disease; the drug has obligatory negative inotropic effects that may not be well tolerated in patients with severe left ventricular dysfunction.

I.V verapamil and I.V diltiazem

They are calcium channel blockers that are less easily titrated than esmolol but nonetheless provide rapid slowing of the ventricular rate in SVT within minutes. The agents are therapeutically equivalent for purposes of AV nodal blockade

I.V diltiazem has less negative inotropic action

Digitalis, diltiazem and Amiodaron it is preferable in patients with heart failure.

Patients with congestive heart failure

It must be temporarily supplemented with other agents because of its slow onset about 6 h.

I.V. digoxin slows the ventricular response during SVT through its vagotonic effects.

- Paroxysmal SVT (PSVT) due to re-entrant circuits that involve accessory pathways such as Wolff±Parkinson±White Syndrome) makes challenge in the management of SVT
- There is risk for developing ventricular ®brillation (VF) upon exposure to classic AV-nodal blocking agents (digoxin, calcium channel blockers, beta blockers, adenosine) because these agents reduce the accessory bundle refractory period.
- I.V. Procainamide, which slows conduction over the accessory bundle, is mandatory option.
- Flecainide and amiodarone should also be considered,
- Cardiology consultation may be helpful
- **Indications for chemical cardioversion of SVT**
    1. Patients cannot tolerate (or do not respond to) rate control therapy,
    2. Failure of DC cardioversion, and remain hemodynamically unstable.
    3. For intraoperative patients who are stable and rate controlled in SVT, First, the 24 h rate of spontaneous conversion to sinus rhythm for recent-onset perioperative SVT exceeds 50%,
    - **Elective DC cardioversion** is considered, it may be mandatory to minimize the risk of SVT recurrence following electrical cardioversion, until the therapeutic

level of an antiarrhythmic agent that maintains sinus rhythm (i.e. procainamide, amiodarone) becomes effective.

- **Ventricular tachycardia**

The management of torsades de pointes differs markedly from other forms of VT, and includes

- I.V magnesium sulfate (2±4 g),
- Increasing the heart rate atropine, isoprenolol .
- Temporary atrial or ventricular pacing.
- Hemodynamic collapse with torsades requires asynchronous DC counter shocks.
- Start ALS.

Antiarrhythmic therapy

- Agents devoid of K+ -channel blocking properties such as lidocaine or phenytoin are usually chosen to avoid further prolongation of the QT interval.
- I.V lidocaine, the putative Na+ -channel blocker most often used during intraoperative cardiac arrest, promotes the conversion of sustained VT or VF to sinus rhythm in any setting
- Magnesium and Na+ -channel blocking agents may be administered empirically.

- **IV Amiodaron**
- o It is an alternative therapy for refractory polymorphic VT of unclear aetiology..
- o It has non-competitive alpha- and beta-blocking effects.
- o rapid i.v. loading may exacerbate hemodynamic instability during the initial (rapid) loading phase in patients with severe left ventricular dysfunction systemic
- o Initial bolus pressers to maintain perfusion.
- The risk of proarrhythmic events may be increased by the simultaneous use of more than one antiarrhythmic agent, and should be avoided if possible.

- . Recent recommendations by the American Heart Association have therefore changed the recommendation for lidocaine to `indeterminate', below amiodarone and procainamide

Acute heart failure:

Causes of acute heart failure in old Eisenmenger syndrome in non cardiac surgery:

1. Myocardial ischemia or infarction.
2. Worsening of cardiac valve dysfunction.
3. Atrial fibrillation and other arrhythmias.
4. Cardio toxic agents.
5. Stress-induced (Takotsubo) cardiomyopathy.
6. Rapid progression of underlying chronic HF.
7. Noncardiac precipitants include severe hypertension, renal failure, and pulmonary emboli.
8. Fluid overload (eg, due to blood transfusion).

Considerations apply to treatment of ADHF in patients presenting with acute coronary syndromes

American College of Cardiology/American Heart Association(ACC/AHA) ST elevation MI guidelines published in the 2004 with 2007 focused update, the
2007 ACC/AHA unstable angina/non-ST elevation MI guideline, and the 2009 focused update of the 2005 ACC/AHA HF guideline

i. Urgent Revisualization
ii. Medical treatment

- Diuretic use
- Supplemental oxygen
- Morphine sulfate
- Vasodilator therapy
- Beta blocker therapy

- ACE inhibitor and ARB therapy
- Aldosterone antagonists
- Management of low input state
- Inotropic agents
- Dopamine
- Dobutamine

Risk of bleeding includes:

- Limitation of anticoagulation to urgent indications for anticoagulation such as atrial fibrillation, recurrent thromboembolism events, mechanical heart valve prostheses;
- The optimal range of the INR or aPTT has not been evaluated. Recommendations for therapeutic anticoagulation are a target INR between 2.0 and 2.5 (in the absence of a mechanical valve) or a therapeutic aPTT of 1.5 times of the normal value;
- Prompt therapy of respiratory tract infections.
- Use of air filters in all intravenous lines.
- Intravenous pacemaker or ICD systems are contraindicated as transvenous leads are associated with a 2-fold increased risk of systemic thromboembolism in patients with intracardiac shunts.

Fluid management in patient of Eisenmenger syndrome

Aim

Achieve an optimal value of stroke volume should be used where possible as this may reduce postoperative complication rates and duration of hospital stay. This may be supplemented by a low dose dopexamine infusion.

Factors controlling fluid management in patient of Eisenmenger syndrome

- **Surgical stress response**
- Surgery elicits a stress response of combined endocrine and inflammatory origin. The hormonal release in response to surgical trauma therefore generally induces a shift toward water and sodium retention, while the excretion of potassium is increased, paralleling the increase in catabolism.
- Several of the hormones involved in this response may exert a potentially on the distribution of body fluids .endocrine response to surgical trauma leads to conservation of sodium and water and to excretion of potassium
- Antidiuretic hormone (ADH), aldosterone and the renin±angiotensin II system.
- The increased ADH secretion leads to enhanced water reabsorption in the kidney, resulting in a postoperative decrease in diuresis and a decrease in plasma concentrations of sodium.
- The increased secretion of aldosterone and rennin leads to conservation of sodium and excretion of potassium.
- Surgical stress,, increased cortical secretion, an obligatory stress response.
- Atrial Natriuretic peptide (ANP) secretion in response to surgery is unclear because ANP secretion may be increased in older patients, in contrast to unchanged ANP levels in younger patients.
- ANP may induce Natriuretic, diuresis and inhibition of aldosterone and ADH secretion. Inflammatory mediators, like IL-6, TNF, substance-P and bradykinin may act as vasodilators and increase capillary permeability. The release of these inflammatory mediators is proportional to the magnitude of the surgical trauma

  - Avoid of dehydration as increases risk of thrombosis and thernbo-embolism and renal impairment.

Fluid overload effects
- On Cardiac functions
  Increased demands on cardiac function, due to an excessive shift to the right on the Starling myocardial performance curve, may potentially increase postoperative cardiac morbidity

- Pulmonary function

  Fluid accumulation in the lungs may predispose patients to pneumonia and respiratory failure

- Recovery of gastrointestinal motility (postoperative ileus) .Gastrointestinal motility may be inhibited, prolonging postoperative ileus and translocation of endotoxin or bacteria, with potentially deleterious implications such as sepsis and multiorgan failure.

- Tissue oxygenation Excess fluid may decrease tissue oxygenation with implications for wound (anastomotic) healing

- Coagulation may be enhanced with crystalloids

- Renal effects

  The excretory demands of the kidney are increased, and the resulting diuresis may lead to urinary retention mediated by the inhibitory effects of anesthetics and analgesics on bladder function

Fluid therapy in cardiac surgery patients should be managed according to predefined target parameters.

Target parameters: • SzvO2 > 70% o. SvO2>65% • MAP>65mmHg • CVP: 8-12mmHg • CI>2.0 l/min/m2 • PAOP: 12-15mmHg • Diuresis> 0, 5 ml/kgBW/h

crystalloid solutions are applied, full electrolytes preparations should be preferred.

- HES and gelatin products
- Human albumin may be used as colloid solutions.

Cardiac surgery clinicians use artificial colloid solutions, mainly applying middle-molecular hydroxyethylene starch derivatives, followed by crystalloid solutions

Recommendation for fluid management

Preoperative treatment with intravenous fluid and inotropes should be aimed at achieving predetermined goals for cardiac output and oxygen delivery as this may improve survival

Hypovolemia

Diagnosis of hypovolemia

Clinically on the basis of pulse, peripheral perfusion and capillary refill,

Venous (JVP/CVP) pressure

Glasgow Coma Scale

Acid-base and lactate measurements

A low urine output can be misleading

Monitoring of the volume status

- The response to a bolus infusion of 200 ml of a suitable colloid or crystalloid should be tested. The response should be assessed using the patient's cardiac output and stroke volume measured by flow-based technology if available.

- Clinical response may be monitored by measurement/estimation of the pulse, capillary refill, CVP and blood pressure before and 15 minutes after receiving the infusion. This procedure should be repeated until there is no further increase in stroke volume and improvement in the clinical parameters.

- trans-esophageal 19 Doppler or pulse contour analysis

- fluid therapy guided by measurements of stroke volume and cardiac index result in significantly better clinical outcomes than those associated with traditional intraoperative monitoring

- The volume and type of fluids given perioperatively should be reviewed and compared with fluid losses in theatre including urine and insensible losses.

- Postoperative treatment with intravenous fluid and low dose dopexamine should be considered, in order to achieve a predetermined value for systemic oxygen delivery, as this may reduce postoperative complication rates and duration of hospital stay.

- When patient in border hear failure, and edematous correction of hypovolemia by gradual persistent negative sodium and water balance based on urine sodium concentration or excretion. Plasma potassium concentration should be monitored and where necessary potassium intake adjusted especially if there are digoxin and Frusemide taken.

- Hypovolemia due predominantly to blood loss should be treated with either a balanced crystalloid solution or a suitable colloid until packed red cells are available.
- Patients to excrete excess sodium and water are compromised, placing them at risk of severe interstitial edema. The administration of large volumes of colloid without sufficient free water (e.g. 5% dextrose) may precipitate a hyperoncotic state.

Renal protection during hypovolemia

- Treatment of hypovolemia in surgical patients impaired renal function due to Eisenmenger syndrome or in due to decrease renal function in elderly patient should follow similar principles to those outlined for patients with normal renal function.
- those patients have reduced capacity to excrete fluid and electrolytes.
- Excessive administration of salt and water will result in interstitial edema and a greater risk of developing hyperkalaemia.
- Early referral to the renal team is recommended to help with clinical evaluation of the patient's volume status and appropriate fluid management. fluids containing potassium to patients with impaired kidney functions due to the risks of precipitating hyperkalaemia.
- Ringer's lactate has been demonstrated to be safe for plasma volume expansion in patients undergoing renal transplantation.
- patients receiving 0.9% saline had an increased incidence of metabolic acidosis and hyperkalaemia

- It is certainly important to prescribe adequate crystalloid when administering colloid solutions to avoid inducing a hyperoncotic state.

- In patients who show signs of refractory fluid overload, renal replacement therapy should be considered early to mobilize interstitial edema and correct extracellular electrolyte and acid base abnormalities.

Management of Hypervolemia in Eisenmenger syndrome:

    Hypervolemia can precipitate to acute heart failure.

    Factor may affect the treatment of Hypervolemia:

        a. Renal protection by continuous renal perfusion

        b. Hypotension with the risk of right to left shunt

Management of fluid overload in Eisenmenger syndrome

Diuretics

- Intravenous (i.v.) administration of loop diuretics is recommended as a first-line treatment
- they rapidly decrease the ventricular filling pressure, reduce pulmonary congestion, and relieve from dyspnea
- Adverse events, especially when used in high doses (>80 mg of I.V. Frusemide).
- They activate the neurohormonal system and indirectly deteriorate the function of the left ventricle
- Significant electrolyte abnormalities (e.g. hypokalaemia)
- Potential arrhythmias.
- ototoxicity (when administered in high IV. doses
- Increase systemic vascular resistance,
- plasma rennin and aldosterone activity,
- Plasma levels of neurohormonal.
- They result in deterioration of renal function and increase of the mortality risk.

Different precipitating factors decrease diuretic response

- decreased intestinal absorption of oral diuretics due to mucosal edema
- impaired renal perfusion,
- decreased diuretic excretion into the urine (due to hypertrophy of distal tubular epithelial cells
- inadequate drug dosing, excess salt intake,

- The concomitant use of NSAIDs.
- This effect could be overdriven with a continuous infusion of furosemide
- a second diuretic agent (e.g. an i.v. thiazide diuretic),
- cause sequential nephron blockade of sodium reabsorption
- Combination therapy requires may lead to excessive sodium and potassium loss.

Factors reduce renal function affection:

- Evaluation extreme clinical conditions, such as cardiogenic shock or acute renal failure.
- Started on the lowest dose of an ACE inhibitor.
- Management of dehydration.
- Avoid concomitant use of NSAIDs should be avoided.
- Titration of dosage should be done very gradually and carefully.
- Close monitoring of hemodynamic and kidney functions.
- Continue these agents during Decompensation, unless renal dysfunction is steadily impaired and severe hyperkalaemia develops.

Dopamine

- Dopamine is an endogenous catecholamine that acts on a variety of receptors (renal, splanchnic, cardiac, vascular) according to the dose infusedit used as infusion at low doses (≤ 3 μg/kg/min),
- The mechanism of action it selectively stimulates receptors in the renal and splanchnic vasculature, increasing blood flow in these tissues.
- it attenuates the effects of norepinephrine and aldosterone

Dobutamine, Milirinone

It is positive inotropic drugs include beta-adrenergic agonists

Inortops should be restricted only to circulatory collapse states, for short term and under close monitoring, as they are susceptible to malignant arrhythmogenesis and loss of myocardial cells by ischemia or apoptosis. They lead to increased myocardial oxygen demand in a period of myocardial energy depletion. It has been shown that in both acute and chronic HF.

Mechanism of action

Phosphodiesterase inhibitors increase levels of cyclic adenosine monophosphate (cAMP), resulting in increased levels of calcium ions within the cardiac myocyte and increased cardiac contractility.

Indication for their use

- ADHF

- Peripheral hypoperfusion (hypotension, deterioration of renal function, cutaneous signs of poor peripheral perfusion)

- Refractoriness to diuretics and vasodilators

- inotropic agents, compared with placebo and vasodilators, have been related to an increased risk of death..

Levosimendan

- Levosimendan is a new inotropic agent novel class of 'calcium sensitizers'.

- It improve symptoms of congestion, and in improve central haemodynamic parameters in patients hospitalized with low cardiac output syndrome.

Mechanism of action

1. It binds to cardiac troponine C, stabilizing the conformational alteration of troponine C through binding to calcium, therefore improving cross-bridging and contractility

2. It also stimulates peripheral vasodilatation through activation of adenosine triphosphate (ATP)-sensitive potassium channels of vascular smooth muscle cells. As it has a neutral effect on cAMP levels

Vasodilators

IV nitroglycerin is recommended for the first-line treatment of ADHF associated with elevated systemic blood pressure at presentation.

They are much less harmful to kidney function, especially when used at low doses that do not cause hypotension and hypoperfusion.

Mechanism of action

- Vasodilators can rapidly reduce ventricular filling pressures and central venous pressures and reduce myocardial oxygen consumption.

- I.V. nitroglycerine is a vasodilator used to improve pulmonary congestion and dyspnea in patients with ADHF.

- Frequent dose titration according to systemic blood pressure to achieve the desired hemodynamic effects.

- Tolerance for The use of continuous i.v. administration of nitrates is associated,

- The reduction in venous pressure may be beneficial in decreasing transrenal perfusion pressure.

B-type Natriuretic peptide (BNP)

- Nesritide, a recombinant human B-type atrial Natriuretic peptide, is an effective vasodilator with a mild diuretic action.

- It is formed in the ventricular myocardium in response to overload and wall stress. BNP causes dilation of both arteries and veins, enhances sodium renal excretion, and suppresses the RAAS.

- It is the only vasodilator recently approved in the USA for the treatment of AHF

Ularatide

- Ularitide is a synthetic form of urodilatin; it is related to family of atrial Natriuretic peptides.

- Urodilatin is synthesized in renal distal tubular cells and plays an important role in sodium and water excretion.

Relaxin

- Relaxin is a natural peptide that was first identified as a reproductive hormone.

- It plays a major role in the hemodynamic and renal adjustments that occur during pregnancy.

Mechanism of action

- The actions of Relaxin include the production of NO, VEGF, matrix metallo proteinases, and inhibition of endothelin and angiotensin II. These actions promote systemic and renal vasodilatation and increased arterial compliance.

Ultrafiltration
- ultra filtration is more efficient in removing sodium, while the neurohormonal activation is less for the same degree of volume reduction
- Ultra filtration slightly influences the patients' hemodynamics parameters.
- The volume of water removed per ultra filtration session is 3–4 lt.
- The reduction in water is accompanied by decreases in right atrial pressure and wedge pressure.
- Cardiac output and stroke volume do not change or rise slightly.

Criteria for the initiation of mechanical fluid removal
1. pulmonary edema with significant renal dysfunction (creatinine clearance <30 ml/min),
2. marked volume overload in patients with ADHF, including significant dysfunction of the right ventricle

3. Refractoriness to IV. Diuretics status.
4. Moreover, the fluid removal volumes and rates are adjustable and weight loss is sustained relatively to Frusemide treatment. Loop diuretics should not be administered during the ultrafiltration sessions, so as to minimize electrolyte abnormalities and further neurohormonal activation.

Cardiocirculatory mechanical support

Indications
- Extra-corporeal membrane oxygenation (ECMO) is instituted for the management of life-threatening pulmonary
- cardiac failure (or both)

- No other treatment has been successful.
- treatment of cardiogenic shock
- Improvement of peripheral perfusion.
- can be used as a bridge to a more permanent device (e.g. BiVAD) or cardiac transplantation

Heart failure

Cause of heart failure in Eisenmenger in elderly patient

i. Decompensation of pre-existing chronic heart failure (e.g. cardiomyopathy)

ii. Acute coronary syndromes (a) myocardial infarction/unstable angina with large extent of ischemia and ischemic dysfunction (b) mechanical complication of acute myocardial infarction (c) right ventricular infarction

iii. Hypertensive crisis

iv. Acute arrhythmia (ventricular tachycardia, ventricular fibrillation, atrial fibrillation or flutter, other supraventricular tachycardia)

v. Valvular regurgitation

vi. Severe aortic valve stenosis

vii. Acute severe myocarditis

viii. Non-cardiovascular precipitating factors

o infections, particularly pneumonia or septicaemia   severe brain insult
o after major surgery
o reduction in renal function
o asthma
o drug abuse
o alcohol abuse
o anemia

Killips classification.

Stage I: No heart failure. No clinical signs of cardiac decompensation;

Stage II: Heart failure. Diagnostic criteria include rales, S3 gallop and pulmonary venous hypertension.

Pulmonary congestion with wet rales in the lower half of the lung fields;

Stage III: Severe heart failure, Frank pulmonary edema with rales throughout the lung fields.

Stage IV: Cardiogenic shock. Signs include hypotension (SBP 90mmHg), and evidence of peripheral vasoconstriction such as Oliguria, cyanosis and diaphoresis.

Clinical evaluation

- Evaluation from the central jugular venous pressure.
- When the internal jugular veins are impractical for evaluation (e.g. due to venous valves) the external jugular veins can be used. Caution is necessary in the interpretation of high measured central venous pressure (CVP) in AHF, as this may be a reflection of decreased venous compliance together with decreased RV compliance even in the presence of low RV filling.

Left sided failure is assessed by chest auscultation, with the presence of wet rales in the lung fields usually indicating raised pressure. The confirmation, classification of severity, and clinical follow-up of pulmonary congestion and pleural effusions should be done using the chest X-ray.

ECG

The ECG may also indicate acute right or left ventricular or atrial strain, perimyocarditis and pre-existing conditions such as left and right ventricular hypertrophy or dilated cardiomyopathy. Cardiac arrhythmia should be assessed in the 12-lead ECG as well as in continuous ECG monitoring.

Chest X-ray

Evaluate pre-existing chest or cardiac conditions (cardiac size and shape) and to assess pulmonary congestion. It is used both for confirmation of the diagnosis, and for follow-up of improvement or unsatisfactory response to therapy.

Chest X-ray allows the differential diagnosis of left heart failure from inflammatory or infectious lung diseases.

Chest CT scan with or without contrast angiography and scintigraphy may be used to clarify the pulmonary pathology and diagnose major pulmonary embolism.

CT scan or transesophageal echocardiography should be used in cases of suspicion of aortic dissection

Labs

Electrolytes, creatinine, and glucose or markers for infection or other metabolic disorders should be done. Hypo– or hyperkalaemia must be controlled.

Management of acute heart failure

- Immediate resuscitation ALS, BLS.
- If the patient is distressed or in pain ,analgesia and sedation
- Arterial oxygen less than 95% increase FIO2, CPAP, and NIPV.
- Treatment of abnormal heart rate and rhythm by pacing ,and treatment of arrhythmias
- Adequate fluid preload cautiously.
- If mean blood pressure more than 77 mmHg give vasodilator (nitroprusside, NTG consider inotrope (dobutamine, levosimendan, PDEI), diuretics in volume overload.
- If there is no adequate cardiac output, metabolic acidosis, SVO2 is less than 65% consider inotropes, or afterload management.

General therapeutic approach in AHF by findings on invasive hemodynamic monitoring

Executive summary of the guidelines on the diagnosis and treatment of acute heart failure The Task Force on Acute Heart Failure of the European Society of Cardiology European Heart Journal (2005) 26, 384–416 doi:10.1093/eurheartj/ehi044

CI, PCWP. SBP,   decreased   consider fluid
Decrease, normal, increased,   SBP more than 85 vasodilator, fluid
load

Decrease, high, less than 85mmHg diuretics	inotrpes dobutamine and dopamine iv
Decreased, high more than 85 vasodialator IV.	inotropes , levosimendan, PDEI
	Diuretics

Maintained ,high IV diuretics If SBP is low, vasoconstrictive, inotropes

Positioning and Eisenmenger syndrome

Prone positioning

- Prone positioning decreases blood pressure and cardiac function.

- The changes in cardiac function after prone positioning are linked to reduced venous return and ventricular compliance.

- Adequate fluid replacement reduced hypotension and hemodynamic instability after prone positioning. The prone position caused left ventricular volume to decrease.

- The prone position also led to decreased systolic pulmonary venous flow velocity and pulmonary venous velocity time integral and enhancement of diastolic pulmonary venous flow velocity and pulmonary venous velocity time integralI.

- These changes were probably due to a decrease in the venous return due to inferior vena caval compression, and decreased left ventricular compliance due to increased intrathoracic pressure in the prone position. .

- The Jackson spine table and longitudinal bolsters had minimal effects on cardiac function, and should be considered in patients with limited cardiac reserve

Trendelenburg position

- Trendelenburg **position** caused only a slight increase of preload volume, despite marked increases in cardiac-filling pressures, without significantly improving cardiac performance.

- The Trendelenburg position in awake and anesthetized patients increased pulmonary arterial pressures (PAP), central venous pressure (GVP) and pulmonary capillary wedge pressure (PCWP), and decreased cardiac output.

Post operative management:

Postoperative care

1. **monitoring**

- Eisenmenger pts be observed in an intensive care unit overnight.

- Eisenmenger pts should be observed on a monitored bed ,ventricular and supraventricular tachycardia, bradyarrhythmia, and myocardial ischemia

2. **Prevent venous stasis**

- Early ambulation

- Applying effective elastic stocking or periodic pneumatic compression.

3. Prevent hypovolemia fluid balance is essential.

4. Change position slowly until the risk of postoperative postural hypotension with secondary increase in right to left shunting.

5. **Postoperative Pain control**

Postoperative pain can result in adverse hemodynamics and possibly hypercoagulable state

It has been suggested that patient-controlled analgesia techniques are associated with greater pt satisfaction and lower pain scores.

Precautions during postoperative pain control

- However, most analgesics can cause a drop in afterload and, more right to left shunting in Eisenmenger syndrome.

- Unstable hemodynamics and the altered mental status .

6. **Inotropic support**

7. **Mechanical ventilation**

8. **Nutritional support**: Surgical patients should be nutritionally screened, and NICE guidelines for perioperative nutritional support should be taken to mitigate risks of the refeeding syndrome.

Case study

Case of female patient 78 year old with long standing Eisenmenger syndrome had future neck femur, arthroplasty under hemi spinal anesthesia .after one month recurrence of fractures, hemiarthroplasty under hemi spinal anesthesia again.

Preoperative preparation

History

A 78 year old female was admitted with fracture left neck of femur for hemiarthroplasty operation. The patient is known case of congenital heart disease. No history of dyspnea, orthopnea , paroxysmal nocturnal dyspnea, syncope, chest pain or stroke .There is history of lower limb oedema treated with furosemide 20 mg once daily and tablet digoxin 0.25 µg daily.

Physical examination

On examination blood pressure 120/60, heart rate 100 irrigular, congested neck veins up to the angle of the mandible. There are central cyanosis, bilateral clubbing of upper and lower limb with no lower limb oedema. Chest examination is free.Cardiac examination revealed Dexrocardia, harsh pansystolic murmur over the right parasternal area. Another pansystolic murmur over the apex of the heart propagating to the right axilla was osculated.

Investigations before the first operation:

Electrocardiogram showed atrial fibrillation rate 105 per minute, right bundle branch block and poor progression of 'R' wave in V1-V leads. Chest x-ray obtained unremarkable.

ECHO cardiography showed: ejection fraction 57%, Dextrocardia, large VSD 1.4cm with right to left shunt with systolic pressure gradient 70 mmHg, moderate to severe TR, moderate MR, dilated and hypertrophied RV with preserved systolic function, hugely dilated right atrium, severe pulmonary hypertension with pulmonary artery systolic pressure 125 mmHg.

Laboratory investigations: Complete blood picture, renal and liver function tests, coagulation profile abdominal ultrasonography were within normal limits, Na and k, exclude hypokalmia and digoxin toxicity.

Preoperative preparation:

The patient started Sildanfil therapy 25mg tablets every 12 hours for three days preoperative.

Frusemide 20 mg once daily and tablet digoxin 0.25 µg treatment was taken before operation.

Ampicillin and gentamicin were administered for prophylaxis against bacterial endocarditis.

An 18G intravenous canula was inserted and secured in left hand vein and left external jugular vein 16G canula was inserted.

Dc shock prepared for uneventful dysarrethemias.

Intraoperative management:

Monitoring:

ECG leads, non invasive blood pressure, pulse oximeter were attached for continuous monitoring. Right internal jugular vein triple lumen central venues line was inserted under local anesthesia.

20G Arterial canula was inserted and secured in left radial artery after modified Allens test for invasive blood pressure monitoring.

The baseline parameters were pulse rate: 100/ min, BP: 110/70 mm Hg   SpO2 87% on oxygen by facemask. central venus pressure was 10 cm H_2O.

Anesthesetic management:

After preloading with 250 ml of Ringer solution, patient was positioned in left lateral position. Spinal anesthesia was done, spinal needle 22G was inserted in L4-5 interspace under comlete aseptic precautions after local infiltration of skin with 2% lignocaine. We injected 2 ml of 0.5% bupivacaine heavy and 25 microgram fentanyl.

Intraoperative events

Patient developed hypotension (90/50) (a fall of more than 20% of the baseline level) at 5 min after institution of spinal anesthesia, and it was successfully treated with bolus doses of injection 6 mg ephedrine each and titrated intravenous Ringer's solution. Pressure was maintained in same range throughout the procedure. Central venous pressure was maintained 10 cm water with ringer solution. The surgical procedure was done in lateral position and was completed in 50 minutes; The total fluid output was 600cc urine and 500cc blood.

500cc crystalloids, 250 ml of blood and two units of fresh frozen plasma were infused to the patient.

After surgery, the patient was transported to intensive care unit for continuous hemodynamic and SpO_2 monitoring with oxygen via a face mask. Postoperative ECHO cardiology was as before surgery.

On the third day post operative the patient suffered from an attack of convulsion which lasted for 1minute followed by disturbed level of consciousness the patient was put on mechanical ventilator CT brain was done with no abnormalities. 12hours later the patient regained consciousness. Subsequent recovery was uneventful and satisfactory. The patient was discharged from the hospital on 10th day postoperative.

After one month recurrence of fracture occurred again repeating investigation revealed the same as first time, Preoperative and intraoperative management was the same as the first operation.

Intraoperative events were:

Hypoxia developed with oxygen saturation87% and was rapidly managed by oxygen face mask.

another attack of hypotension was developed (90/50) after institution of spinal anesthesia, and it was successfully treated with bolus doses of injection 6 mg ephedrine each and titrated intravenous Ringer's solution. Postoperative recovery was satisfactory. The patient was discharged from the hospital on 10th day postoperative.

Discussion

A primary goal of anesthetic management in this case is to minimize increases in pulmonary vascular resistance and to maintain systemic vascular resistance. Abrupt increases in pulmonary vascular resistance may precipitate either acute right ventricular failure or oxygen desaturation followed by decreased cardiac output. Severe bradycardia may occur with progression to cardiac arrest.

Prevention and treatment of pulmonary hypertensive crisis includes hyperventilation, correction of acidosis, avoidance of sympathetic nervous system stimulation, maintenance of normothermia, minimization of intrathoracic pressure, and use of inotropic support.

Regional anesthesia may be an acceptable alternative to general anesthesia. However, spinal may produce unacceptable decreases in systemic vascular resistance in patients, and this action could exacerbate right to left shunting.

We chose to do low dose spinal anesthesia to decreases afterload, prevented myocardial depression. Fluid management is also critical and preloading the patient in the preoperative period is not desirable because it may precipitate a congestive heart failure. In our case fluid overloading was prevented by titrate the fluids to maintain a CVP of 10 cm H2O. Invasive blood pressure monitoring and central venous pressure monitoring were used to facilitate early recognition of blood pressure changes and to guide fluid therapy and maintain normovolemia..

The major risks during the intraoperative and postoperative period are similar to the risks described above. These risks include bleeding, dysrhythmias, and thromboembolic events, oral pulmonary vasodilatators such as Sildanfil may be beneficial (15).

Similar case study was done by B. Ghai, V. Mohan, M. Khetarpal andN. Malhotra(16). They reported the anesthetic management for cesarean section of a 27-year-old multigravid female at 35 weeks' gestation with Eisenmenger syndrome. Titrated epidural anesthesia was administered with incremental doses of 2% lidocaine. Intraoperative course was uneventful except for an episode of hypotension immediately after delivery of the baby, which was managed successfully. they conclude that carefully titrated epidural anesthesia may be effective for patients with Eisenmenger's syndrome for cesarean section.

Robert S. Holzman, Charles D. Nargozian, Richard Marnach, Curtis O. McMillan **(17)** presented two cases of patients with palliated cyanotic congenital heart disease received Epidural anesthesia. the first case is A 17.year-old, 54kgs boy with a d-transposition of the great arteries, hypoplastic right ventricle , ventricular septal defect (atrioventricular canal type), atrial septal defect, small patent ductus arteriosus, and an overriding tricuspid valve The patient took digoxin and Frusemide he presented for a right inguinal herniorrhaphy. The second one is a 30-year-old, 50-kg woman with a history of tetralogy of Fallot with pulmonary atresia, an interatrial communication, and large aortopuhnonary collaterals presented for exploratory laparotomy for excision of an ovarian cyst. The patient took tetracycline, digoxin, and Frusemide. Prior surgical procedures included a central shunt, left pleurectomy, odontectomy, and bilateral tubal ligation. Surgery proceeded uneventfully once anesthesia was established; Surgery lasted for 75 minutes in patient 1, and 50 minutes in patient 2.

In astudy of Martin JT et al (18) , they had a literature identified 57 articles describing 103 anesthetics in patients with Eisenmenger syndrome. An additional 21 anesthetics were identified in patients receiving regional anesthesia for labor,theu found that Overall perioperative mortality was 14%; patients receiving regional anesthesia had a mortality of 5%, whereas those receiving general anesthesia had a mortality of 18%. This trend favored the use of regional anesthesia but was not statistically significant. A better predictor of outcome was the nature of the surgery (and presumably the surgical disease). Patients requiring major surgery had mortality of 24%, whereas those requiring minor surgery had mortality of 5% (P <.05). Patients in labor receiving regional anesthesia had a mortality rate of 24%, and most of these occurred several hours after delivery. They concluded that most deaths probably occurred as a result of the surgical procedure and disease and not anesthesia. Although perioperative and peripartum mortalities are high, many anesthetic agents and techniques have been used with success.

In another study of Gurumurthy,etal(19) ,he published a case of 22-year-old primigravida weighing 46 kg, known case of Eisenmenger syndrome at 37 weeks of gestation, was scheduled for an elective caesarean section. At the age of 15 years, a cardiac catheterization was performed, which revealed a large mid-muscular VSD with severe pulmonary arterial hypertension (120/50 mmHg). She was explained about the existing cardiac condition and advised to avoid strenuous work.

They concluded that although pregnancy must be discouraged in women with Eisenmenger's syndrome, it can be successful. Safe anaesthetic management of these patients requires meticulous preparation and familiarity with all the anaesthetic agents to maintain the cardiovascular stability. Then, early extubation should be avoided in such patients because, invariably, they may go for worsening of shunt and thrombo embolic phenomena as these complications can occur as late as the third post-operative day, as seen in our patient and other reports. they recommended a general anaesthetic technique with maintenance of haemodynamics as close to normal as possible, with adequate control of pain and early initiation of thromboprophylaxis for successful management of similar cases .Another case study for Lipi Mishra,etal (20),they described a case of a pregnant patient with a large ventricular septal defect (VSD) and pulmonary artery hypertension, presented to the hospital and underwent elective cesarean section under epidural anesthesia and postoperative analgesia. The procedure was uneventful till the patient was discharged on 10(th) day

Conclusion

When an elderly patient with long standing Eisenmenger syndrome needs an emergency anesthesia for hemiarthroplasty the anesthetic management becomes a challenge. Proper understanding of the Pathophysiology of the disorder and Careful anesthesia planning, pre-operative assessment, intraoperative and postoperative management can help in reducing the mortality. Low-dose intrathecal bupivacaine and fentanyl provided the advantages of spinal and should be under invasive cardiovascular monitoring.

References

1. Mitchell SC, Korones SB, Berendes HW: Congenital heart disease in 56,109 births. Incidence and natural history. Circulation 1971; 43:323–32Mitchell, SC Korones, SB Berendes,

2. , Hansen PB, Søndergaard L (April 2009). "[Eisenmenger syndrome]". *Ugeskrift for Laeger (in Danish) 171 (15): 1270–5. PMID 19416617.*

3. "Eisenmenger syndrome" at *Dorland's Medical Dictionary*

4. *Siddiqui S, Latif N (2008). "PGE1 nebulisation during caesarean section for Eisenmenger's syndrome: a case report". J Med Case Reports 2 (1): 149.*

5. Braunwald E. Heart Disease: A Textbook of Cardiovascular Medicine. P 1617-1618. Ann Intern Med 1998; 128:745-755

6. *"Eisenmenger syndrome". NIH MedLine Plus. 2010-02-0*

7. Sorbini CA, Grassi V, Solinas E, Muiesan G. Arterial oxygen tension in relation to age in healthy subjects.Respiration. 1968;25:3–13.

8. Miller R. Miller's Anesthesia. 6th ed. Churchill Livingstone; 2004.

9. Ergina PL, Gold SL, Meakins JL. Perioperative care of the elderly patient. World J Surg. 1993;17:192–198.

10. Amar D, Zhang H, Leung DH, Roistacher N, Kadish AH. Older age is the strongest predictor of postoperative atrial fibrillation. Anesthesiology. 2002;96:352–356.

11. Grandison MK, Boudinot FD. Age-related changes in protein binding of drugs: implications for therapy.Clin Pharmacokinet. 2000;38:271–290.

12. Kudravi SA, Reed MJ. Aging, cancer and wound healing. In Vivo. 2000;14:83–92.

13. Kirkbride DA, Parker JL, Williams GD, Buggy DJ. Induction of anesthesia in the elderly ambulatory patient: a double-blinded comparison of propofol and sevoflurane. Anesth Analg. 2001;93:1185–1187.[PubMed]

14. Maxime Cannesson, M.D.; Michael G. Earing, M.D.; Vincent Collange, M.D.;Judy R. Kersten, M.D., F.A.C.C. Anesthesia for Noncardiac Surgery in Adults with Congenital Heart Disease Anesthesiology 8 2009, Vol.111, 432-440.

15. Ghai B[1], Mohan V, Khetarpal M, Malhotra N.Epidural anesthesia for cesarean section in a patient with Eisenmenger's syndrome Int J Obstet Anesth. 2002 Jan;11(1):44-7.

16. Holzman RS[1], Nargozian CD, Marnach R, McMillan CO..Epidural anesthesia in patients with palliated cyanotic congenital heart diseaseJ Cardiothorac Vasc Anesth. 1992 Jun;6(3):340-3

17. Martin JT[1], Tautz TJ, Antognini JF: Safety of regional anesthesia in Eisenmenger's syndrome. Reg Anesth Pain Med. 2002 Sep-Oct;27(5):509-13.

18. Gurumurthy T[1], Hegde R, Mohandas B :Anaesthesia for a patient with Eisenmenger's syndrome undergoing caesarean section Indian J Anaesth. 2012 May;56(3):291-4. doi: 10.4103/0019-5049.98780.

19. Lipi Mishra, Nibedita Pani, Ramesh Samantaray, and Kalyani Nayak: Eisenmenger's syndrome in pregnancy: Use of epidural anesthesia and analgesia for elective cesarean section J Anaesthesiol Clin Pharmacol. 2014 Jul;30(3):425-6.

20. Sear JW[1], Higham H.Issues in the perioperative management of the elderly patient with cardiovascular disease. Drugs Aging. 2002;19(6):429-51.

21. Bellomo R, Kellum JA, Ronco C: Defining and classifying acute renal failure: From advocacy to consensus and validation of the RIFLE criteria. Intensive Care Med 2007; 33: 409 – 413 19

22. Hoste EA, Clermont G, Kersten A, et al: RIFLE criteria for acute kidney injury are associated with hospital mortality in critically ill patients: A cohort analysis. Crit Care 2006; 10:R73

23. George H. Crossley, MD, FHRS,1 Jeanne E. Poole, MD, FHRS,2 Marc A. Rozner, PhD, MD,3 * Samuel J. Asirvatham, MD, FHRS,4 Alan Cheng, MD,5! Mina K. Chung, MD, FHRS,6 T. Bruce Ferguson, Jr., MD,7## John D. Gallagher, MD,8 * Michael R. Gold, MD, PhD, FHRS,9# Robert H. Hoyt, MD,10 Samuel Irefin, MD,11* Fred M. Kusumoto, MD, FHRS,12 Liza Prudente Moorman, MSN, ACNP, FHRS,13 Annemarie Thompson, MD14*The Heart Rhythm Society (HRS)/American Society of Anesthesiologists (ASA) Expert Consensus Statement on the Perioperative Management of Patients with Implantable Defibrillators, Pacemakers and Arrhythmia Monitors: Facilities and Patient Management: Executive Summary This document was developed as a joint project with the American Society of Anesthesiologists (ASA), and in collaboration with the American Heart Association (AHA), and the Society of Thoracic Surgeons (STS) Lee D,

Sharp VJ, Konety BR. Use of bipolar power source for transurethral resection of bladder tumor in patient with implanted pacemaker. Urology 2005;66: 194.

24. Bayes J. A survey of opthalmic anesthetists on managing pacemakers and implanted cardiac defibrillators. Anesth Analg 2010;103:1615–1616.

25. Belott PH, Sands S, Warren J. Resetting of DDD pacemakers due to EMI. Pacing Clin Electrophysiol 1984;7:169 –172.

26. Domino KB, Smith TC. Electrocautery-induced reprogramming of a pacemaker using a precordial magnet. Anesth Analg 1983;62:609 – 612.

27. Godin JF, Petitot JC. STIMAREC report. Pacemaker failures due to electrocautery and external electric shock. Pacing Clin Electrophysiol 1989;12:1011.

28. Heller LI. Surgical electrocautery and the runaway pacemaker syndrome. Pacing Clin Electrophysiol 1990;13:1084 –1085.

29. Irnich W, de Bakker JM, Bisping HJ. Electromagnetic interference in implantable pacemakers. Pacing Clin Electrophysiol 1978;1:52– 61.

30. . Levine PA, Balady GJ, Lazar HL, Belott PH, Roberts AJ. Electrocautery and pacemakers: management of the paced patient subject to electrocautery. Ann Thorac Surg 1986;41:313–317.

31.

32. Lichner I, Borrie J, Miller WM. Radio-frequency hazards with cardiac pacemakers. Br Med J 1965;1:1513–1518.

33. Mangar D, Atlas GM, Kane PB. Electrocautery-induced pacemaker malfunction during surgery. Br J Anaesth 1991;38:616 – 618.

34. Pfeiffer D, Tebbenjohanns J, Schumacher B, Jung W, Luderitz B. Pacemaker function during radiofrequency ablation. Pacing Clin Electrophysiol 1995; 18(5 Pt 1):1037–1044.

35. Smith RB, Wise WS. Pacemaker malfunction from urethral electrocautery. JAMA 1971; 218:256.

36. Vanerio G, Maloney J, Rashidi R, et al. The effects of percutaneous catheter ablation on preexisting permanent pacemakers. Pacing Clin Electrophysiol 1990;13(12 Pt 1):1637–1645.

37. Wilson JH, Lattner S, Jacob R, Stewart R. Electrocautery does not interfere with the function of the automatic implantable cardioverter defibrillator. Ann Thorac Surg 1991; 51:225–226.

38. Thompson1 and J. R. Balser1 :Perioperative cardiac arrhythmias A. Br J Anaesth 2004; 93: 86±94

39. Amar D, Fogel DH, Shah JP. The Shaw hemostatic scalpel as an alternative to electrocautery in patients with pacemakers. Anesthesiology 1996;85:223.

40. Lamas GA, Antman EM, Gold JP, Braunwald NS, Collins JJ. Pacemaker backup-mode reversion and injury during cardiac surgery. Ann Thorac Surg 1986;41:155–157.

41. Pinski SL, Trohman RG. Interference in implanted cardiac devices, part I. Pacing Clin Electrophysiol 2002; 25:1367–1381.

42. Furman S, Fisher JD. Endless loop tachycardia in an AV universal [DDD] pacemaker. Pacing Clin Electrophysiol 1982;5:486 – 489.

43. Katzenberg CA, Marcus FI, Heusinkveld RS, Mammana RB. Pacemaker failure due to radiation therapy. Pacing Clin Electrophysiol 1982;5:156 –159.

44. Snow JS, Kalenderian D, Colasacco JA, Jadonath RL, Goldner BG, Cohen TJ. Implanted devices and electromagnetic interference: case presentations and review. J Invasive Cardiol 1995;7:25–32.

45. 23. Fiek M, Dorwarth U, Durchlaub I, et al. Application of radiofrequency energy in surgical and interventional procedures: are there interactions with ICDs? Pacing Clin Electrophysiol 2004;27:293–298.

46. Casavant D, Haffajee C, Stevens S, Pacetti P. Aborted implantable cardioverter defibrillator shock during facial electrosurgery. Pacing Clin Electrophysiol 1998;21:1325–1326.

47. Hoyt R, Johnson W, Lieserwitz A. Monopolar electrosurgery interactions with the implantable cardioverter-defibrillator. Heart Rhythm 2010;7:S2.

48. Burke MC, Knight BP. Management of implantable pacemakers and defibrillators at the time of noncardiac surgery. ACC Current Journal Review 2005;14(1): 52–5.

49. Rasmussen MJ, Friedman PA, Hammill SC, Rea RF. Unintentional deactivation of implantable cardioverter-defibrillators in health care settings. Mayo Clin Proc 2002;77:855– 859.

50. Glikson M, Trusty JM, Grice SK, Hayes DL, Hammill SC, Stanton MS. Importance of pacemaker noise reversion as a potential mechanism of pacemakerICD interactions. Pacing Clin Electrophysiol 1998;21:1111–1121.

51. Anonymous. LATITUDE patient management system. Boston Scientific, 2008.

52. American Society of Anesthesiologists Task Force on Perioperative Management of Patients with Cardiac Rhythm Management Devices. Practice advisory for the perioperative management of patients with cardiac rhythm management devices: pacemakers and implantable cardioverter-defibrillators: a report by the American Society of Anesthesiologists Task Force on Perioperative Management of Patients with Cardiac Rhythm Management Devices. Anesthesiology 2005;103:186 –198.

53. Cohan L, Kusumoto F, Goldschlager N. Environmental effects on cardiac pacing systems. Cardiac Pacing Clinician 2008;595– 618.

54. Covidien I. Principles of Electrosurgery Online. 2009. Available at http://www.valleylab.com/education/poes/index.html.

55. Altamura G, Bianconi L, Lo BF, et al. Transthoracic DC shock may represent a serious hazard in pacemaker dependent patients. Pacing Clin Electrophysiol 1995;18(1 Pt 2):194 –198.

56. Waller C, Callies F, Langenfeld H. Adverse effects of direct current cardioversion on cardiac pacemakers and electrodes Is external cardioversion contraindicated in patients with permanent pacing systems? Europace 2004; 6:165–168.

57. Manegold JC, Israel CW, Ehrlich JR, et al. External cardioversion of atrial fibrillation in patients with implanted pacemaker or cardioverter-defibrillator systems: a randomized comparison of monophasic and biphasic shock energy application. EurHeart J 2007;28:1731–1738.

58. Falk RH, Battinelli NJ. External cardiac pacing using low impedance electrodes suitable for defibrillation: a comparative blinded study. J Am Coll Cardiol 1993;22:1354 –1358.

59. Lakkireddy D, Patel D, Ryschon K, et al. Safety and efficacy of radiofrequency energy catheter ablation of atrial fibrillation in patients with pacemakers and implantable cardiac defibrillators. Heart Rhythm 2005;2:1309 – 1316.

60. Ellenbogen KA, Wood MA, Stambler BS. Acute effects of radiofrequency ablation of atrial arrhythmias on implanted permanent pacing systems. Pacing Clin Electrophysiol 1996;19:1287–1295.

61. McCollough CH, Zhang J, Primak AN, Clement WJ, Buysman JR. Effects of CT irradiation on implantable cardiac rhythm management devices. Radiology 2007;243:766 –774.

62. Yamaji S, Imai S, Saito F, Yagi H, Kushiro T, Uchiyama T. Does high-power computed tomography scanning equipment affect the operation of pacemakers? Circ J 2006;70:190 –197.

63. Adamec R, Haefliger JM, Killisch JP, Niederer J, Jaquet P. Damaging effect of therapeutic radiation on programmable pacemakers. Pacing Clin Electrophysiol 1982; 5:146 –150.

64. A. Reuter a1, T.

W. Felbinger a1, C. Schmidt a1, K. Moerstedt a1, E. Kilger a1,P. Lamm a2 and A. E. Goetz Trendelenburg positioning after cardiac surgery: effects on intrathoracic blood volume index and cardiac performance European Journal of Anaesthesiology / Volume / Issue 01 / January 2003, pp 17-20

65. Brooks C, Mutter M. Pacemaker failure associated with therapeutic radiation. Am J Emerg Med 1988; 6:591–593? 43. Allergan. Directions for Use: Style 133V Series Tissue Expander Matrix with Magna-Site Injection Sites. Allergan, 2008

66. Schoeck AP, Mellion ML, Gilchrist JM, Christian FV. Safety of nerve conduction studies in patients with implanted cardiac devices. Muscle Nerve 2007;35: 521–524.

67. LaBan MM, Petty D, Hauser AM, Taylor RS. Peripheral nerve conduction stimulation: its effect on cardiac pacemakers. Arch Phys Med Rehabil 1988;69: 358 –362

68. Drach GW, Weber C, Donovan JM. Treatment of pacemaker patients with extracorporeal shock wave lithotripsy: experience from 2 continents. J Urol 1990;143:895– 8

69. Hall MJ, Owings MF. 2000 National Hospital Discharge Sur-vey. Hyattsville, MD: Department of Health and Human Ser-vices; 2002. Advance Data From Vital and Health Statistics,No. 329

70. 2. Goldman L,Caldera D,Nussbaum S, et al. Multifactorial index ofcardiac risk in noncardiac surgical procedures. N Engl J Med 1977;297:845

71. Eagle KA, Berger PB, Calkins H, et al. ACC/AHA guideline update for perioperative cardiovascular evaluation for noncar-diac surgery-executive summary. A report of the American Col-lege of Cardiology / American Heart Association Task Force onPractice Guidelines (Committee to update the 1996 guidelineson Perioperative Cardiovascular Evaluation for Noncardiac Sur-gery). Anesth Analg 2002; 94:1052.

72. Detsky AS, Abrams HB, Forbath N , et al. Cardiac assessmentfor patients undergoing noncardiac surgery. A multifactorial clini-cal risk index. Arch Intern Med 1986; 146:2131.

73. Eagle K, Brundage B, Chaitman B, et al. Guidelines forperioperative cardiovascular evaluation for non-cardiac surgery. AHA/ACC task force report. J Am Coll Cardiol 1996; 27:910.

74. Stoelting RK, Dierdorf S. Ischemic heart disease. In:Stoelting RK, Dierdorf S, editors. Anesthesia and co-existing disease. The edition. Philadelphia. Churchill Livingstone 2002. p.2-8.

75. London MJ, Zaugg M, Schaub MC, et al. Perioperative beta-adrenergic receptor blockade: physiologic foundations and clini-cal controversies. Anesthesiology 2004; 100:170.

76. Dupuis JY, Labinaz M. Noncardiac surgery in patients withcoronary artery stent : what should the anaesthesiologist know? Can J Anaesth 2005;52:356.

77. Barash PG.Sequential monitoring of myocardial ischemia in theperioperative period.In: American Society of AnaesthesiologistsReview Lectures.Atlanta: American Society ofAnaesthesiology;2005.p.411.

78. Breen P, Park K W. General anesthesia versus regional anesthe-sia. Int Anesthesiol Clin 2002; 40:61.

79. Bonow RO, Carabello B, de Leon AC Jr, et al. Guidelines for the management of patients with valvular heart disease: Executive summary: a report of the American College of Cardiology / Ameri-can Heart Association Task Force on Practice Guidelines (com-mittee on management of patients with valvular heart disease).Circulation 1998;98:1949-84.

80. Baum VC, Perloff JK. Anesthetic implications of adults with congenital heart disease. Anesth Analg.1993;76:1342–58. [PubMed]

81. Ammash NM, Connolly HM, Abel MD, Warnes CA. Noncardiac surgery in Eisenmenger syndrome. J Am Coll Cardiol. 1999;33:222–7. [PubMed]

82. Diller GP, Dimopoulos K, Broberg CS, et al. Presentation, survival prospects, and predictors of death in Eisenmenger syndrome: a combined retrospective and case-control study. European Heart Journal.2006;27(14):1737–42

83. Lumley J, Whitwam JG, Morgan M. General anesthesia in the presence of Eisenmenger's syndrome.Anesth Analg. 1977;56:543–7. [PubMed]

84. Vongpatanasin W, Brickner ME, Hillis D, Lange RA. The Eisenmenger's syndrome in adult. The Annals of Internal Medicine. 1998;128(9):745–55

85. Foster J., Jones R.M.; The anesthetic management of the Eisenmenger syndrome. Ann R Coll Surg Engl. 66 1984:353-355.

86. Devitt J., Noble W., Byrick R.; A Swan-Ganz catheter related complication in a patient with Eisenmenger's syndrome. Anesthesiology. 57 1982:335-337.

87. Roizeu M.F., Berger D.L., Gerson J.; Practice guidelines for pulmonary artery. A report by the American Society of Anesthesiologists Task Force on Pulmonary Artery Catheterization. Anesthesiology. 78 1993:380-394.

88. Bennett JM[1], Ehrenfeld JM[2], Markham L[3], Eagle SS[2].Anesthetic management and outcomes for patients with pulmonary hypertension and intracardiac shunts and Eisenmenger syndrome: a review of institutional experience. J Clin Anesth. 2014 Jun;26(4):286-93. doi: 10.1016/j.jclinane.2013.11.022. Epub 2014 Jun 6.

89. Antman EM, Anbe DT, Armstrong PW, et al. ACC/AHA guidelines for the management of patients with ST-elevation myocardial infarction. www.acc.org/qualityandscience/clinical/statements.htm (Accessed on August 24, 2006).

90. Antman, E, Hand, M, Armstrong PW, et al. 2007 Focused update of the ACC/AHA 2004 guidelines for the management of patients with ST-elevation myocardial infarction. Available at: www.acc.org/qualityandscience/clinical/statements.htm (accessed May 2, 2008).

91. Anderson JL, Adams CD, Antman EM, et al. ACC/AHA 2007 guidelines for the management of patients with unstable angina/non-ST-Elevation myocardial infarction: a report of the American College of Cardiology/American Heart Association Task Force on Practice Guidelines (Writing Committee to Revise the 2002 Guidelines for the Management of Patients With Unstable Angina/Non-ST-Elevation Myocardial Infarction) developed in collaboration with the American College of Emergency Physicians, the Society for Cardiovascular Angiography and Interventions, and the Society of Thoracic Surgeons endorsed by the American Association of Cardiovascular and Pulmonary Rehabilitation and the Society for Academic Emergency Medicine. J Am Coll Cardiol 2007; 50:e1.

92. Hunt SA, Abraham WT, Chin MH, et al. 2009 focused update incorporated into the ACC/AHA 2005 Guidelines for the Diagnosis and Management of Heart Failure in Adults: a report of the American College of Cardiology Foundation/American Heart Association Task Force on Practice Guidelines: developed in collaboration with the International Society for Heart and Lung Transplantation. Circulation 2009; 119:e391.

93. Rosenzweig EB, Kerstein D, Barst RJ. Long-term prostacyclin for pulmonary hypertension with associated congenital heart defects. *Circulation*. 1999 Apr 13. 99(14):1858-65. [Medline].

94. Fernandes SM, Newburger JW, Lang P, Pearson DD, Feinstein JA, Gauvreau K, et al. Usefulness of epoprostenol therapy in the severely ill adolescent/adult with Eisenmenger physiology. *Am J Cardiol*. 2003 Mar 1. 91(5):632-5. [Medline].

95. Ivy DD, Doran A, Claussen L, Bingaman D, Yetman A. Weaning and discontinuation of epoprostenol in children with idiopathic pulmonary arterial hypertension receiving concomitant bosentan. *Am J Cardiol*. 2004 Apr 1. 93(7):943-6. [Medline]. [Full Text].

96. Ivy DD, Claussen L, Doran A. Transition of stable pediatric patients with pulmonary arterial hypertension from intravenous epoprostenol to intravenous treprostinil. *Am J Cardiol*. 2007 Mar 1. 99(5):696-8. [Medline].[Full Text].

97. Ivy DD, Doran AK, Parker DK, et al. Acute and Chronic Effects of Inhaled Iloprost Therapy in Children with Pulmonary Arterial Hypertension. *Chest*. 2006. 130 (4) Meeting abstracts:156S.

98. Ivy DD, Doran AK, Smith KJ, et al. Short- and long-term effects of inhaled iloprost therapy in children with pulmonary arterial hypertension. *J Am Coll Cardiol*. 2008 Jan 15. 51(2):161-9. [Medline]. [Full Text].

99. Barst RJ, Ivy D, Dingemanse J, et al. Pharmacokinetics, safety, and efficacy of bosentan in pediatric patients with pulmonary arterial hypertension. *Clin Pharmacol Ther*. 2003 Apr. 73(4):372-82. [Medline].

100.   Maiya S, Hislop AA, Flynn Y, Haworth SG. Response to bosentan in children with pulmonary hypertension.*Heart*. 2006 May. 92(5):664-70. [Medline]. [Full Text].

101.   Rosenzweig EB, Ivy DD, Widlitz A, et al. Effects of long-term bosentan in children with pulmonary arterial hypertension. *J Am Coll Cardiol*. 2005 Aug 16. 46(4):697-704. [Medline].

102.   Kaya MG, Lam YY, Erer B, et al. Long-term effect of bosentan therapy on cardiac function and symptomatic benefits in adult patients with Eisenmenger syndrome. *J Card Fail*. 2012 May. 18(5):379-84.[Medline].

103.   Christensen DD, McConnell ME, Book WM, Mahle WT. Initial experience with bosentan therapy in patients with the Eisenmenger syndrome. *Am J Cardiol*. 2004 Jul 15. 94(2):261-3. [Medline].

104.   Schulze-Neick I, Gilbert N, Ewert R, et al. Adult patients with congenital heart disease and pulmonary arterial hypertension: first open prospective multicenter study of bosentan therapy. *Am Heart J*. 2005 Oct. 150(4):716. [Medline].

105.   Galiè N, Beghetti M, Gatzoulis MA, et al. Bosentan therapy in patients with Eisenmenger syndrome: a multicenter, double-blind, randomized, placebo-controlled study. *Circulation*. 2006 Jul 4. 114(1):48-54.[Medline].

106.   Gatzoulis MA, Beghetti M, Galiè N, Granton J, Berger RM, Lauer A, et al. Longer-term bosentan therapy improves functional capacity in Eisenmenger syndrome: results of the BREATHE-5 open-label extension study. *Int J Cardiol*. 2008 Jun 23. 127(1):27-32. [Medline].

107.   Adriaenssens T, Delcroix M, Van Deyk K, Budts W. Advanced therapy may delay the need for transplantation in patients with the Eisenmenger syndrome. *Eur Heart J*. 2006 Jun. 27(12):1472-7.[Medline].

108.   Chau EM, Fan KY, Chow WH. Effects of chronic sildenafil in patients with Eisenmenger syndrome versus idiopathic pulmonary arterial hypertension. *Int J Cardiol*. 2007 Sep 3. 120(3):301-5. [Medline].

109.   Humpl T, Reyes JT, Holtby H, Stephens D, Adatia I. Beneficial effect of oral sildenafil therapy on childhood pulmonary arterial hypertension: twelve-month clinical trial of a single-drug, open-label, pilot study.*Circulation*. 2005 Jun 21. 111(24):3274-80. [Medline].

110.   Raja SG, Danton MD, MacArthur KJ, Pollock JC. Effects of escalating doses of sildenafil on hemodynamics and gas exchange in children with pulmonary hypertension and congenital cardiac defects. *J Cardiothorac Vasc Anesth*. 2007 Apr. 21(2):203-7. [Medline].

111.   Singh TP, Rohit M, Grover A, Malhotra S, Vijayvergiya R. A randomized, placebo-controlled, double-blind, crossover study to evaluate the efficacy of oral sildenafil therapy in severe pulmonary artery hypertension.*Am Heart J*. 2006 Apr. 151(4):851.e1-5. [Medline].

112.   Mukhopadhyay S, Sharma M, Ramakrishnan S, et al. Phosphodiesterase-5 inhibitor in Eisenmenger syndrome: a preliminary observational study. *Circulation*. 2006 Oct 24. 114(17):1807-10. [Medline].

113.   Ivy DD, Griebel JL, Kinsella JP, Abman SH. Acute hemodynamic effects of pulsed delivery of low flow nasal nitric oxide in children with pulmonary hypertension. *J Pediatr*. 1998 Sep. 133(3):453-6. [Medline].

114.   Ivy DD, Parker D, Doran A, Parker D, Kinsella JP, Abman SH. Acute hemodynamic effects and home therapy using a novel pulsed nasal nitric oxide delivery system in children and young adults with pulmonary hypertension. *Am J Cardiol*. 2003 Oct 1. 92(7):886-90. [Medline].

115.   Kinsella JP, Parker TA, Ivy DD, Abman SH. Noninvasive delivery of inhaled nitric oxide therapy for late pulmonary hypertension in newborn infants with congenital diaphragmatic hernia. *J Pediatr*. 2003 Apr. 142(4):397-401. [Medline].

116.   [Guideline] Wilson W, Taubert KA, Gewitz M, et al. Prevention of infective endocarditis: guidelines from the American Heart Association: a guideline from the American Heart Association Rheumatic Fever, Endocarditis, and Kawasaki Disease Committee, Council on Cardiovascular Disease in the Young, and the Council on Clinical Cardiology, Council on Cardiovascular Surgery and Anesthesia, and the Quality of Care and Outcomes Research Interdisciplinary Working Group. *Circulation*. 2007 Oct 9. 116(15):1736-54.[Medline].

117.   [Guideline] Nishimura RA, Carabello BA, Faxon DP, et al. ACC/AHA 2008 guideline update on valvular heart disease: focused update on infective endocarditis: a report of the American College of Cardiology/American Heart Association Task Force on Practice Guidelines: endorsed by the Society of Cardiovascular Anesthesiologists, Society for Cardiovascular Angiography and Interventions, and Society of Thoracic Surgeons. *Circulation*. 2008 Aug 19. 118(8):887-96. [Medline].

118.   Dajani AS, Taubert KA, Wilson W, et al. Prevention of bacterial endocarditis. Recommendations by the American Heart Association. *Circulation*. 1997 Jul 1. 96(1):358-66. [Medline].

119.   Linderkamp O, Klose HJ, Betke K, et al. Increased blood viscosity in patients with cyanotic congenital heart disease and iron deficiency. *J Pediatr*. 1979 Oct. 95(4):567-9. [Medline].

120.   Van De Bruaene A, Delcroix M, Pasquet A, et al. Iron deficiency is associated with adverse outcome in Eisenmenger patients. *Eur Heart J*. 2011 Nov. 32(22):2790-9. [Medline].

121.   Silversides CK, Granton JT, Konen E, Hart MA, Webb GD, Therrien J. Pulmonary thrombosis in adults with Eisenmenger syndrome. *J Am Coll Cardiol*. 2003 Dec 3. 42(11):1982-7. [Medline].

122.   Asling J, Fung D. Epidural anesthesia in Eisenmenger's syndrome: a case report. Anesth Analg; Curr Res 1974;53:965-8.

123.   Perioperative venous thromboembolic disease and the emerging role of the novel oral anticoagulants: An analysis of the implications for perioperative management Martina Mookadam, Fadi E. Shamoun1 , Harish Ramakrishna1 , Hiba Obeid2 , Renee L. Rife3 , Farouk Mookadam1 Department of Family Medicine, 1 Division of Cardiovascular Diseases, 3 Mayo Pharmacy, Mayo Clinic, Scottsdale, Arizona, 2 St. John Hospital and Medical Centers, Detroit, Michigan, USA 2015 Annals of Cardiac Anaesthesia | Published by Wolters Kluwer – Medknow

124.   28. Practice alert for the perioperative management of patients with coronary artery stents: a report by the American Society of Anesthesiologists Committee on Standards and Practice Parameters.*Anesthesiology*. 2009;110:22-23.

125.   Douketis JD, Berger PB, Dunn AS, et al. The perioperative management of antithrombotic therapy: American College of Chest Physicians Evidence-Based Clinical Practice Guidelines (8th Edition).*Chest*. 2008;133:299S-339S.

126.   Gombotz H, Rumpold-Seitlinger F. Volumenersatz in der Herzchirurgie. In: Bold J (Hrsg.) Volumenersatztherapie (S. 187-204). Stuttgart: Georg Thieme Verlag, 2001 2. Zickmann B. Kardiochirurgie. In: Kochs E, Krier C, Buzello W, HA Adams (Hrsg.) Anästhesiologie. AINS Band 1 (S. 1090- 1136). Stuttgart: Georg Thieme Verlag, 2001 3. Stephens R, Mythen M. Optimizing intraoperative fluid therapy. Current Opinion in Anaesthesiology 2003; 16: 385-392 4.

127.   Adams HA. Volumen und Flüssigkeitsersatz – Physiologie, Pharmakologie und klinischer Einsatz. Anästh Intensivmed 2007; 48: 448-60 5.

128.   Guyton AC, Hall JE. The Kidneys and body fluids. In: Guyton AC, Hall JE (Eds.) Textbook of medical physiology (9. ed., pp. 297-312). Philadelphia: WB Saunders Company, 1996 6. Rackow EC, Falk JL, Fein IA, Siegel JS, Packman MI, Haupt MT, Kaufmann BS, Putnam D. Fluid resuscitation in circulatory shock: a comparison of the

cardiorespiratory effects of albumin, hetastarch, and saline solutions in patients with hypovolemic and septic shock. Crit Care Med 1983; 11: 839-850 7.

129.   Boldt J, Kling B, Bormann B von, Hempelmann G. Präoperative normovolämische Hämodilution in der Herzchirurgie. Pulmonale Veränderungen bei Anwendung neuer Techniken. Anästhesist 1989; 38: 294-301 8.

130.   Waters JH, Gottlieb A, Schoenwald P, Popovich MJ, Sprung J, Nelson DR. Normal saline versus lactated Ringer's solution for intraoperative fluid management in patients undergoing abdominal aortic aneurysm repair: an outcome study. Anesth Analg 2001; 93: 817-22 9.

131.   Carl M, Alms A, Braun J, Dongas A, Erb J, Goetz A, Gopfert M, Gogarten W, Grosse J, Heller A, Heringlake M, Kastrup M, Kroner A, Loer S, Marggraf G, Markewitz A, Reuter M, Schmitt DV, Schirmer U, Wiesenack C, Zwissler B, Spies C; German Society for Thoracic and Cardiovascular Surgery; German Society of Anaesthesiology and Intensive Care Medicine. Guidelines for intensive care in cardiac surgery patients: haemodynamic monitoring and cardio-circulatory treatment guidelines of the German Society for Thoracic and Cardiovascular Surgery and the German Society of Anaesthesiology and Intensive Care Medicine Thorac Cardiovasc Surg 2007; 55:130-48

132.   Adams H, Baumann G, Cascorbi I et al. Zur Diagnostik und Therapie der Schockformen. Empfehlungen der interdisziplinären Arbeitsgruppe Schock der DIVI - Teil II: Hypovolämischer Schock. Anästh Intensivmed 2005; 42: 96-109 11.

133.   Kastrup M, Markewitz A, Spies C, Carl M, Erb J, Grosse J, Schirmer U. Current practice of hemodynamic monitoring and vasopressor and inotropic therapy in post-operative cardiac surgery patients in Germany: results from a postal survey. Acta Anaesthesiol Scand 2007; 51: 347-58

134.   O'Malley CM, Frumento RJ, Hardy MA, Benvenisty AI, Brentjens TE, Mercer JS, et al. A randomized, double-blind comparison of lactated Ringer's solution and 0.9% NaCl during renal transplantation. Anesth Analg 2005;100:1518- 1524. 2.

135.   Reid F, Lobo DN, Williams RN, Rowlands BJ, Allison SP. (Ab)normal saline and physiological Hartmann's solution: a randomized double-blind crossover study. Clin Sci (Lond) 2003;104:17-24. 3.

136.   Wilkes NJ, Woolf R, Mutch M, Mallett SV, Peachey T, Stephens R, et al. The effects of balanced versus saline-based hetastarch and crystalloid solutions on acid-base and electrolyte status and gastric mucosal perfusion in elderly surgical patients. Anesth Analg 2001;93:811-816. 4.

137.   Williams EL, Hildebrand KL, McCormick SA, Bedel MJ. The effect of intravenous lactated Ringer's solution versus 0.9% sodium chloride solution on serum osmolality in human volunteers. Anesth Analg 1999;88:999-1003. 5.

138.   Ho AM, Karmakar MK, Contardi LH, Ng SS, Hewson JR. Excessive use of normal saline in managing traumatized patients in shock: a preventable contributor to acidosis. J Trauma 2001;51:173-177. 6.

139.   Waters JH, Gottlieb A, Schoenwald P, Popovich MJ, Sprung J, Nelson DR. Normal saline versus lactated Ringer's solution for intraoperative fluid management in patients undergoing abdominal aortic aneurysm repair: an outcome study. Anesth Analg 2001;93:817-822. 7.

140.   Lobo DN, Bostock KA, Neal KR, Perkins AC, Rowlands BJ, Allison SP. Effect of salt and water balance on recovery of gastrointestinal function after elective colonic resection: a randomised controlled trial. Lancet 2002;359:1812- 1818. 8.

141.   MacKay G, Fearon K, McConnachie A, Serpell MG, Molloy RG, O'Dwyer PJ. Randomized clinical trial of the effect of postoperative intravenous fluid restriction on recovery after elective colorectal surgery. Br J Surg 2006;93:1469-1474. 9.

142.   Beck CE. Hypotonic versus isotonic maintenance intravenous fluid therapy in hospitalized children: a systematic review. Clin Pediatr (Phila) 2007;46:764- 770. 10.

143.   Steele A, Gowrishankar M, Abrahamson S, Mazer CD, Feldman RD, Halperin ML. Postoperative hyponatremia despite near-isotonic saline infusion: a phenomenon of desalination. Ann Intern Med 1997;126:20-25.

144.   Brady M, Kinn S, Stuart P. Preoperative fasting for adults to prevent perioperative complications. Cochrane Database Syst Rev 2003:CD004423. 14. Pre-operative Assessment: The Role of the Anaesthetist. London: The Association of Anaesthetists of Great Britain and Ireland, 2001.

145.   Hausel J, Nygren J, Lagerkranser M, Hellstrom PM, Hammarqvist F, Almstrom C, et al. A carbohydrate-rich drink reduces preoperative discomfort in elective surgery patients. Anesth Analg 2001;93:1344-1350.

146.   Hausel J, Nygren J, Thorell A, Lagerkranser M, Ljungqvist O. Randomized clinical trial of the effects of oral preoperative carbohydrates on postoperative nausea and vomiting after laparoscopic cholecystectomy. Br J Surg 2005;92:415-421.

147.   Noblett SE, Watson DS, Huong H, Davison B, Hainsworth PJ, Horgan AF. Preoperative oral carbohydrate loading in colorectal surgery: a randomized controlled trial. Colorectal Dis 2006;8:563-569.

148.   Soop M, Carlson GL, Hopkinson J, Clarke S, Thorell A, Nygren J, et al. Randomized clinical trial of the effects of immediate enteral nutrition on metabolic responses to major colorectal surgery in an enhanced recovery protocol. Br J Surg 2004;91:1138-1145.

149.   Lobo SM, Salgado PF, Castillo VG, Borim AA, Polachini CA, Palchetti JC, et al. Effects of maximizing oxygen delivery on morbidity and mortality in high-risk surgical patients. Crit Care Med 2000;28:3396-3404.

150.   Sinclair S, James S, Singer M. Intraoperative intravascular volume optimisation and length of hospital stay after repair of proximal femoral fracture: randomised controlled trial [see comments]. BMJ 1997;315:909-912.

151.   Mythen MG, Webb AR. Perioperative plasma volume expansion reduces the incidence of gut mucosal hypoperfusion during cardiac surgery. Arch Surg 1995;130:423-429. 30. Gan TJ, Soppitt A, Maroof M, el-Moalem H, Robertson KM, Moretti E, et al. Goal-directed intraoperative fluid administration reduces length of hospital stay after major surgery. Anesthesiology 2002;97:820-826.

152.   Noblett SE, Snowden CP, Shenton BK, Horgan AF. Randomized clinical trial assessing the effect of Doppler-optimized fluid management on outcome after elective colorectal resection. Br J Surg 2006;93:1069-1076.

153.   Wakeling HG, McFall MR, Jenkins CS, Woods WG, Miles WF, Barclay GR, et al. Intraoperative oesophageal Doppler guided fluid management shortens postoperative hospital stay after major bowel surgery. Br J Anaesth 2005;95:634-642.

154.   Venn R, Steele A, Richardson P, Poloniecki J, Grounds M, Newman P. Randomized controlled trial to investigate influence of the fluid challenge on duration of hospital stay and perioperative morbidity in patients with hip fractures. Br J Anaesth 2002;88:65-71

155.   McKendry M, McGloin H, Saberi D, Caudwell L, Brady AR, Singer M. Randomized controlled trial assessing the impact of a nurse delivered, flow monitored protocol for optimisation of circulatory status after cardiac surgery. BMJ 2004;329:258.

156.   Rokyta R, Jr., Novak I. Fluid challenge in patients at risk for fluid loading-induced pulmonary edema. Acta Anaesthesiol Scand 2004;48:69-73. 42.

157.   Gosling P, Rittoo D, Manji M, Mahmood A, Vohra R. Hydroxyethylstarch as a risk factor for acute renal failure in severe sepsis. Lancet 2001;358:581; author reply 582.

158.   Rittoo D, Gosling P, Simms MH, Smith SR, Vohra RK. The effects of hydroxyethyl starch compared with gelofusine on activated endothelium and the systemic inflammatory response following aortic aneurysm repair. Eur J Vasc Endovasc Surg 2005;30:520-524.

159.   Finfer S, Bellomo R, Boyce N, French J, Myburgh J, Norton R. A comparison of albumin and saline for fluid resuscitation in the intensive care unit. N Engl J Med 2004;350:2247-2256

160.   Abbas SM, Hill AG. Systematic review of the literature for the use of oesophageal Doppler monitor for fluid replacement in major abdominal surgery. Anaesthesia 2008;63:44-51.

161.   Walsh SR, Tang T, Bass S, Gaunt ME. Doppler-guided intra-operative fluid management during major abdominal surgery: systematic review and metaanalysis. Int J Clin Pract 2008;62:466-470.

162.   Pearse RM, Belsey J, Cole J, Bennet ED. Effect of dopexamine infusion on mortality following major surgery: Individual patient data meta-regression analysis of published clinical trials. Crit Care Med 2008;36:1323-1329. 52. Walsh SR, Cook EJ, Bentley R, Farooq N, Gardner-Thorpe J, Tang T, et al. Perioperative fluid management: prospective audit. Int J Clin Pract 2008;62:492-497. 53.

163.   Brandstrup B, Tonnesen H, Beier-Holgersen R, Hjortso E, Ording H, LindorffLarsen K, et al. Effects of intravenous fluid restriction on postoperative

complications: comparison of two perioperative fluid regimens: a randomized assessor-blinded multicenter trial. Ann Surg 2003;238:641-648. 54.

164.   Effect of prone positioning systems on hemodynamic and cardiac function during lumbar spine surgery: an echocardiographic study. Spine (Phila Pa 1976). 2006 May 20;31(12):1388-93;

165.   Toyota S[1], Amaki Y.Hemodynamic evaluation of the prone position by transesophageal echocardiography. J Clin Anesth. 1998 Feb;10(1):32-5.

166.   Kita T, Mammoto T, Kishi Y. Fluid management and postoperative respiratory disturbances in patients with transthoracic esophagectomy for carcinoma. J Clin Anesth 2002;14:252-256. 37 55.

167.   Nisanevich V, Felsenstein I, Almogy G, Weissman C, Einav S, Matot I. Effect of intraoperative fluid management on outcome after intraabdominal surgery. Anesthesiology 2005;103:25-32.

168.   Arieff AI. Fatal postoperative pulmonary edema: pathogenesis and literature review. Chest 1999;115:1371-1377.

169.   Lobo DN, Dube MG, Neal KR, Allison SP, Rowlands BJ. Peri-operative fluid and electrolyte management: a survey of consultant surgeons in the UK. Ann R Coll Surg Engl 2002;84:156-160

170.   . Lobo DN, Dube MG, Neal KR, Simpson J, Rowlands BJ, Allison SP. Problems with solutions: drowning in the brine of an inadequate knowledge base. Clin Nutr 2001;20:125-130.

171.   Walsh SR, Walsh CJ. Intravenous fluid-associated morbidity in postoperative patients. Ann R Coll Surg Engl 2005;87:126-130.

172.   Pearse R, Dawson D, Fawcett J, Rhodes A, Grounds RM, Bennett ED. Early goal-directed therapy after major surgery reduces complications and duration of hospital stay. A randomised, controlled trial [ISRCTN38797445]. Crit Care 2005;9:R687-693

173.   . Pearse RM, Dawson D, Fawcett J, Rhodes A, Grounds RM, Bennett D. The incidence of myocardial injury following post-operative Goal Directed Therapy. BMC Cardiovasc Disord 2007;7:10.

174.   Polonen P, Ruokonen E, Hippelainen M, Poyhonen M, Takala J. A prospective, randomized study of goal-oriented hemodynamic therapy in cardiac surgical patients. Anesth Analg 2000;90:1052-1059.

175.   Lobo DN, Bjarnason K, Field J, Rowlands BJ, Allison SP. Changes in weight, fluid balance and serum albumin in patients referred for nutritional support. Clin Nutr 1999;18:197-201.

176.   National Collaborating Centre for Acute Care. Nutrition support in adults Oral nutrition support, enteral tube feeding and parenteral nutrition. London: National Collaborating Centre for Acute Care, 2006. (Also available from: http://www.nice.org.uk/Guidance/CG32, accessed 20 July 2008).

177.   Brunkhorst FM, Engel C, Bloos F, Meier-Hellmann A, Ragaller M, Weiler N, et al. Intensive insulin therapy and pentastarch resuscitation in severe sepsis. N Engl J Med 2008; 358:125-139.

178.   . Cittanova ML, Leblanc I, Legendre C, Mouquet C, Riou B, Coriat P. Effect of hydroxyethylstarch in brain-dead kidney donors on renal function in kidneytransplant recipients. Lancet 1996;348:1620-1622.

179.   Schortgen F, Lacherade JC, Bruneel F, Cattaneo I, Hemery F, Lemaire F, et al. Effects of hydroxyethylstarch and gelatin on renal function in severe sepsis: a multicentre randomised study. Lancet 2001;357:911-916.

180.   Palevsky PM. Clinical review: Timing and dose of continuous renal replacement therapy in acute kidney injury. Crit Care 2007;11:232.

181.   . Sever MS, Vanholder R, Lameire N. Management of crush-related injuries after disasters. N Engl J Med 2006;354:1052-1063.

182.   . Latta T. Malignant cholera. Documents communicated by the Central Board of Health, London, relative to the treatment of cholera by copious injection of aqueous and saline fluids into the veins. Lancet 1832;ii:274-277. 38

183.   . Awad S, Allison SP, Lobo DN. The history of 0.9% saline. Clin Nutr 2008;27:179-188. 72. Evans GH. The abuse of normal salt solution. JAMA 1911;57:2126-2127. 73. Coller FA, Campbell KN, Vaughan HH, Iob LV, Moyer CA. Postoperative salt intolerance. Ann Surg 1944;119:533-541.

184.   Le Quesne LP, Lewis AAG. Postoperative water and sodium retention. Lancet 1953;1:153-158. 75. Moore FD. Metabolic Care of the Surgical Patient. Philadelphia: W. B. Saunders, 1959. 76. Stoneham MD, Hill EL. Variability in post-operative fluid and electrolyte prescription. Br J Clin Pract 1997;51:82-84.

185.   . Zikria BA, Bascom JU. Mechanisms of multiple organ failure. In: Zikria BA, Oz MC, Carlson RW, eds. Reperfusion injuries and clinical capillary leak syndrome. Armonk, NY: Futura, 1994.

186.   Toraman F, Evrenkaya S, Yuce M, Turek O, Aksoy N, Karabulut H, et al. Highly positive intraoperative fluid balance during cardiac surgery is associated with adverse outcome. Perfusion 2004;19:85-91.

187.   Bellomo R, Raman J, Ronco C. Intensive care unit management of the critically ill patient with fluid overload after open heart surgery. Cardiology 2001;96:169-176.

188.   Lobo DN, Macafee DA, Allison SP. How perioperative fluid balance influences postoperative outcomes. Best Pract Res Clin Anaesthesiol 2006;20:439- 455.

189.   Callum KG, Gray AJG, Hoile RW, Ingram GS, Martin IC, Sherry KM, et al. Extremes of Age: The 1999 Report of the National Confidential Enquiry into Perioperative Deaths. London: National Confidential Enquiry into Perioperative Deaths, 1999.

190.   Lobo DN, Stanga Z, Simpson JAD, Anderson JA, Rowlands BJ, Allison SP. Dilution and redistribution effects of rapid 2-litre infusions of 0.9% (w/v) saline and 5% (w/v) dextrose on haematological parameters and serum biochemistry in normal subjects: a double-blind crossover study. Clin Sci (Lond) 2001; 101:173-179.

191.   Maack T. Role of atrial natriuretic factor in volume control. Kidney Int 1996;49:1732-1737.

192.   Lobo DN, Myhill DJ, Stanga Z, Broughton Pipkin F, Allison SP. The effect of volume loading with 1 litre intravenous infusions of 0.9% saline and 5% dextrose on the renin angiotensin system (RAS) and volume controlling hormones: a randomized, double blind, crossover study [abstract]. Clin Nutr 2002;21 (S1):9-10.

193.   Wilcox CS. Regulation of renal blood flow by plasma chloride. J Clin Invest 1983;71:726-735

194.   Roberts I, Alderson P, Bunn F, Chinnock P, Ker K, Schierhout G. Colloids versus crystalloids for fluid resuscitation in critically ill patients. Cochrane Database Syst Rev 2004:CD000567

195.   Traylor RJ, Pearl RG. Crystalloid versus colloid versus colloid: all colloids are not created equal. Anesth Analg 1996;83:209-212. 39

196.   Westphal M, James MF, Kozek-Langenecker S, Guidet B, Van Aken H. Hydroxyethyl starches: different products - different effects. Anesthesiology 2009;111:187-202.

197.   Healey MA, Davis RE, Liu FC, Loomis W, Hoyt DB. Lactated Ringer's is superior to normal saline in a model of massive hemorrhage and resuscitation. J Trauma 1998;45:894-898; discussion 898-899.

198.   Waters JH, Bernstein CA. Dilutional acidosis following hetastarch or albumin in healthy volunteers. Anesthesiology 2000;93:1184-1187.

199.   Skellett S, Mayer A, Durward A, Tibby SM, Murdoch IA. Chasing the base deficit: hyperchloraemic acidosis following 0.9% saline fluid resuscitation. Arch Dis Child 2000;83:514-516.

200.   Allison SP. Metabolic aspects of intensive care. Br J Hosp Med 1974;11:860-871

201.   Allison S. Fluid, electrolytes and nutrition. Clin Med 2004;4:573-578.

202.   Veech RL. The toxic impact of parenteral solutions on the metabolism of cells: a hypothesis for physiological parenteral therapy. Am J Clin Nutr 1986;44:519-551.

203.   Bowyer MW. Fluid therapy. In: Parsons PE, Wiener-Kronish JP, eds. Critical Care Secrets. St. Louis: Mosby Year Book, 1992: 24-26.

204.   Gosling P. Salt of the earth or a drop in the ocean? A pathophysiological approach to fluid resuscitation. Emerg Med J 2003;20:306-315.

205.   Krishna GG, Chusid P, Hoeldtke RD. Mild potassium depletion provokes renal sodium retention. J Lab Clin Med 1987;109:724-730.

206.   Kucuk HF, Cevik A, Kurt N, Bildik N, Gulmen M. [The effects of abdominal compartment syndrome on the serum urea and creatinine levels]. Ulus Travma Derg 2002;8:11-15.

207.   de Cleva R, Silva FP, Zilberstein B, Machado DJ. Acute renal failure due to abdominal compartment syndrome: report on four cases and literature review. Rev Hosp Clin Fac Med Sao Paulo 2001;56:123-130.

208.   Ma YM, Qian C, Xie F, Zhou FH, Pan L, Song Q. Acute renal failure due to abdominal compartment syndrome. Zhonghua Yi Xue Za Zhi 2005;85:2218- 2220.

209.   Stone HH, Fulenwider JT. Renal decapsulation in the prevention of post ischemia oliguria. Ann Surg 1977;186:343-355. 102. Fleck A, Raines G, Hawker F, Trotter J, Wallace PI, Ledingham IM, et al. Increased vascular permeability: a major cause of hypoalbuminaemia in disease and injury. Lancet 1985;1:781-784.

210.   McDonald DM, Thurston G, Baluk P. Endothelial gaps as sites for plasma leakage in inflammation. Microcirculation 1999;6:7-22.

211.   Flear CT, Singh CM. Hyponatraemia and sick cells. Br J Anaesth 1973;45:976-994. 105. Flear CT, Singh CM. The sick cell concept and hyponatremia in congestive heart failure and liver disease. Lancet 1982;2:101-102.

212.   Campbell IT, Green CJ, Jackson MJ. Muscle glycogen and electrolyte concentrations in multiple organ failure [abstract]. Proc Nutr Soc 1998;57:111A. 40

213.   Cunningham JN, Jr., Shires GT, Wagner Y. Changes in intracellular sodium and potassium content of red blood cells in trauma and shock. Am J Surg 1971;122:650-654. 108. Waterlow JC. Protein-energy malnutrition. London: Smith-Gordon and Company, 2006. 109. Moritz ML, Ayus JC. Hospital-acquired hyponatremia--why are hypotonic parenteral fluids still being used? Nat Clin Pract Nephrol 2007;3:374-382.

214.   Yung M, Keeley S. Randomised controlled trial of intravenous maintenance fluids. J Paediatr Child Health 2007.

215.   . Choong K, Kho ME, Menon K, Bohn D. Hypotonic versus isotonic saline in hospitalised children: a systematic review. Arch Dis Child 2006;91:828-835.

216.   Hoorn EJ, Lindemans J, Zietse R. Development of severe hyponatraemia in hospitalized patients: treatment-related risk factors and inadequate management. Nephrol Dial Transplant 2006;21:70-76.

217.   Soupart A, Decaux G. Therapeutic recommendations for management of severe hyponatremia: current concepts on pathogenesis and prevention of neurologic complications. Clin Nephrol 1996;46:149-169.

218.   Lobo DN, Allison SP. Fluid, electrolyte and nutrient replacement. In: Burnand KG, Young AE, Lucas J, Rowlands BJ, Scholefield J, eds. The New Aird's Companion in Surgical Studies. 3rd ed. London: Churchill Livingstone, 2005: 20-41.

219.   Sanders G, Mercer SJ, Saeb-Parsey K, Akhavani MA, Hosie KB, Lambert AW. Randomized clinical trial of intravenous fluid replacement during bowel preparation for surgery. Br J Surg 2001;88:1363-1365. 116. Zmora O, Wexner SD, Hajjar L, Park T, Efron JE, Nogueras JJ, et al. Trends in preparation for colorectal surgery: survey of the members of the American Society of Colon and Rectal Surgeons. Am Surg 2003;69:

220.   154. 117. Lassen K, Hannemann P, Ljungqvist O, Fearon K, Dejong CH, von Meyenfeldt MF, et al. Patterns in current perioperative practice: survey of colorectal surgeons in five northern European countries. BMJ 2005;330:1420-1421.

221.   Allison SP, Lobo DN. Fluid and electrolytes in the elderly. Curr Opin Clin Nutr Metab Care 2004;7:27-33. 119. Pearse RM, Harrison DA, James P, Watson D, Hinds C, Rhodes A, et al. Identification and characterisation of the high-risk surgical population in the United Kingdom. Crit Care 2006;10:R81.

222.   Cullinane M, Gray AJG, Hargraves CMK, Lansdown M, Martin IC, Schubert M. The 2003 Report of the National Confidential Enquiry into Perioperative Deaths. London: National Confidential Enquiry into Perioperative Deaths, 2003.

223.   . Jhanji S, Dawson J, Pearse RM. Cardiac output monitoring: basic science and clinical application. Anaesthesia 2008;63:172-181.

224.   . Kaplan LJ, Frangos S. Clinical review: Acid-base abnormalities in the intensive care unit -- part II. Crit Care 2005;9:198-203.

225.   Wade CE, Grady JJ, Kramer GC, Younes RN, Gehlsen K, Holcroft JW. Individual patient cohort analysis of the efficacy of hypertonic saline/dextran 41 in patients with traumatic brain injury and hypotension. J Trauma 1997;42:S61-65.

226.   Battison C, Andrews PJ, Graham C, Petty T. Randomized, controlled trial on the effect of a 20% mannitol solution and a 7.5% saline/6% dextran solution on increased intracranial pressure after brain injury. Crit Care Med 2005;33:196-202

227.   Wade CE, Kramer GC, Grady JJ, Fabian TC, Younes RN. Efficacy of hypertonic 7.5% saline and 6% dextran-70 in treating trauma: a metaanalysis of controlled clinical studies. Surgery 1997;122:609-616.

228.   . Mythen MG, Webb AR. Intra-operative gut mucosal hypoperfusion is associated with increased post-operative complications and cost. Intensive Care Med 1994;20:99-104.

229.   . Rivers E, Nguyen B, Havstad S, Ressler J, Muzzin A, Knoblich B, et al. Early goal-directed therapy in the treatment of severe sepsis and septic shock. N Engl J Med 2001;345:1368-1377.

230.   . Solomon SM, Kirby DF. The refeeding syndrome: a review. JPEN J Parenter Enteral Nutr 1990;14:90-97.

231.   . Wind J, Polle SW, Fung Kon Jin PH, Dejong CH, von Meyenfeldt MF, Ubbink DT, et al. Systematic review of enhanced recovery programmes in colonic surgery. Br J Surg 2006;93:800-809.

232.   Heyland DK, Dhaliwal R, Drover JW, Gramlich L, Dodek P. Canadian clinical practice guidelines for nutrition support in mechanically ventilated, critically ill adult patients. JPEN J Parenter Enteral Nutr 2003;27:355-373.

233.   Martin CM, Doig GS, Heyland DK, Morrison T, Sibbald WJ. Multicentre, cluster-randomized clinical trial of algorithms for critical-care enteral and parenteral therapy (ACCEPT). CMAJ 2004;170:197-204.

234.   Simpson F, Doig GS. Parenteral vs. enteral nutrition in the critically ill patient: a meta-analysis of trials using the intention to treat principle. Intensive Care Med 2005;31:12-23.

235.   Tellado JM, Garcia-Sabrido JL, Hanley JA, Shizgal HM, Christou NV. Predicting mortality based on body composition analysis. Ann Surg 1989;209:81-87.

236.   Stanga Z, Brunner A, Leuenberger M, Grimble RF, Shenkin A, Allison SP, et al. Nutrition in clinical practice-the refeeding syndrome: illustrative cases and guidelines for prevention and treatment. Eur J Clin Nutr 2008;62:687- 694.

237.   . Chertow GM, Levy EM, Hammermeister KE, Grover F, Daley J. Independent association between acute renal failure and mortality following cardiac surgery. Am J Med 1998;104:343-348.

238.   Praught ML, Shlipak MG. Are small changes in serum creatinine an important risk factor? Curr Opin Nephrol Hypertens 2005;14:265-270.

239.	Sakr Y, Payen D, Reinhart K, Sipmann FS, Zavala E, Bewley J, et al. Effects of hydroxyethyl starch administration on renal function in critically ill patients.